THE
HEALTHY
STUDENT
COOKBOOK

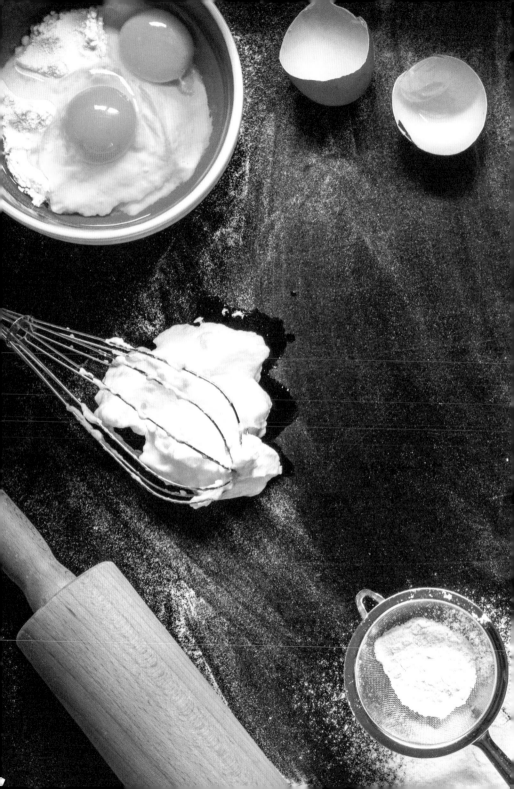

THE HEALTHY STUDENT COOKBOOK

Bounty
Books

An Hachette UK Company
www.hachette.co.uk

First published in Great Britain in 2016 by
Spruce,
a division of Octopus Publishing Group Ltd
Carmelite House
50 Victoria Embankment
London EC4Y 0DZ
www.octopusbooks.co.uk

This edition published in 2017 by Bounty Books,
a division of Octopus Publishing Group Ltd

ISBN 978-0-75373-246-5

A CIP catalogue record for this book is available from the British Library

Printed and bound in China

10 9 8 7 6 5 4 3 2 1

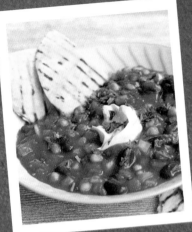

mixed bean and
tomato chilli

The recipes in this book have been labelled if suitable for Gluten Free, Vegan and
Vegetarian diets. Vegetarians should look for the 'V' symbol on a cheese to ensure it is
made with vegetarian rennet. There are vegetarian forms of Parmesan, Feta, Cheddar,
Cheshire, Red Leicester, dolcelatte and many goats' cheeses, among others.

Standard level spoon measurement are used in all recipes.
1 tablespoon = one 15 ml spoon
1 teaspoon = one 5 ml spoon

Both imperial and metric measurements have been given in all recipes. Use one
set of measurements only and not a mixture of both.

Ovens should be preheated to the specific temperature – if using a fan-assisted oven,
follow manufacturer's instructions for adjusting the time and the temperature.

Pepper should be freshly ground black pepper unless otherwise stated.

For the Bounty edition
Publisher: Lucy Pessell
Designer: Lisa Layton
Editor: Sarah Vaughan
Production Controller: Beata Kibil

contents

Introduction 6

Brekky and Lunchbox 12

Healthy and Hearty 40

Super Salads, Snacks
and Sides 104

Sweet Alternatives 138

Back to Basics 162

Index and Acknowledgements 172

Introduction

Leaving home and living on your own for the first time is both challenging and exciting. And while you're settling in, meeting new people and getting to grips with your independence, food can swiftly slide down the list of priorities. But it's important to establish good habits from the beginning and try to incorporate healthy eating as part of a healthy lifestyle. It's no more expensive or time consuming to eat healthily as a student; it just takes a bit more planning. So, if you want to enjoy a varied diet that doesn't have to be emptied on to your plate from a polystyrene tub, it's time to up your game in the kitchen and get to grips with ingredients and cooking techniques.

Cooking for Yourself

Whether you live on campus or in shared accommodation, you'll need to be organized when it comes to budgeting and shopping for food. If you're moving in with people you already know then it makes sense to work out what kitchen equipment you'll need and divide the list between you. That way, you won't end up with six juicers and an empty crockery cupboard. Likewise, when it comes to shopping, your budget will stretch much further if you pool your resources and shop as a household. You can buy ingredients in bulk and make the most of buy-one-get-one-free deals. However, you will need to take individual preferences and diets into account – it's hardly fair if the vegetarian among you has to fund a weekly meat feast.

Foodie Friction

Food can be the cause of tension in shared student houses so it's a good idea to set out a few simple rules when you first move in. That doesn't mean installing CCTV in the fridge and keeping your favourite cereal in a safe in case anyone tries to tuck into a bowl for breakfast. But it does mean working out a cooking and shopping rota, if you're going to eat meals together. You'll need to decide on a feasible weekly food budget and allocate someone to take control of it. You obviously won't all be eating at home every night of the week so you could, for example, club together for midweek meals and then let everyone fend for themselves at the weekend.

Where to shop

The internet makes it easy for a shared household to do their food shop. You can pick a time when everyone is around so you all get to have a say in what makes it into the trolley. A meal planner will make it much easier to shop to budget and if this is agreed in advance, there'll be fewer 'discussions' about which ingredients you need to buy. Shopping online means you don't all have to trek to the supermarket together – a particular drag if no one has a car. You can order your shopping in one go and get it delivered when you know someone will be at home. Local markets and farmers' markets often offer value for money, especially for seasonal produce. This is a great way to shop for a special weekend meal, or local ingredients that you won't see in the supermarket.

Stock up your storecupboard

Your first grocery shop will probably be the most expensive, as you'll need to stock up on storecupboard essentials that form the basis of many meals. Alternatively, as with equipment, you could devise a list and ask everyone to bring a few items when you move in. Here's the lowdown on what you should line your cupboards with on moving-in day.

- **Condiments** Salt and pepper are essential for many recipes and good seasoning will liven up most dishes. You will also need vegetable oil for cooking and olive oil for dressings and sauces. Ketchup, mayonnaise and mustard are also staples.
- **Butter** toast is a student staple so a good supply of butter or margarine is essential. This is also an important ingredient for mash.
- **Spices** You don't need a full range of spices in a student kitchen but if you stock up on chilli powder, turmeric, cumin and maybe some mustard and fennel seeds, you'll be able to rustle up a half decent curry. Stock cubes and bouillon powders are also handy when you don't have any fresh stock made up (see Back to Basics, pages 164–71).
- **Onions and garlic** Like salt and pepper, onion and garlic are vital ingredients in all manner of dishes across all cuisines. These have a long shelf life if you keep them in the fridge.
- **Pasta and rice** Bakes, salads, risottos, curries, soups, pilafs... the list is endless and a good stock of pasta and rice will see you through the lean times.
- **Pulses and grains** Split peas, lentils, couscous, bulgar wheat and quinoa are fantastic storecupboard staples for meals in their own right, or used to bulk up soups and stews.

Cans Cans of beans (kidney beans, butter beans, and so on), sweetcorn and chickpeas are dependable favourites when the budget is suffering. They are cheap and nutritious and can be swiftly turned into a curry or chilli with a few additional ingredients.

Freezer staples A lot of student accommodation suffers from the lack of a decent freezer and you might have to make do with a couple of shelves or a small compartment at the top of the fridge. But as long as there's space for some frozen vegetables and a few tubs of leftovers you should be able to get by.

Healthy week meal planner

	MONDAY	TUESDAY	WEDNESDAY	THURSDAY	FRIDAY	SATURDAY	SUNDAY
BREAKFAST	MANGO & ORANGE SMOOTHIE (page 16)	BERRY, HONEY & YOGURT POTS (page 21)	MIXED GRAIN PORRIDGE (page 25)	MAPLE-GLAZED GRANOLA WITH FRUIT (page 24)	APPLE & YOGURT MUESLI (page 23)	WHOLEMEAL BLUEBERRY PANCAKES WITH LEMON CURD YOGHURT (page 29)	BANANA & SULTANA DROP SCONES (page 26)
LUNCH	TURKEY & AVOCADO SALAD (page 121)	FALAFEL PITTA POCKETS (page 32)	HEARTY MINESTRONE (page 42)	TANDOORI CHICKEN SALAD (page 120)	MUSHROOM & ROCKET SEEDED WRAP WITH FETA & GARLIC DRESSING (page 38)	BAKED SWEET POTATOES (page 72)	SPINACH & POTATO TORTILLA (page 62)
DINNER	SPAGHETTI CARBONARA (page 51)	BAKED COD WITH TOMATOES & OLIVES (page 98)	SMOKED MACKEREL SUPERFOOD SALAD (page 114)	RANCH-STYLE EGGS (page 60)	CAULIFLOWER & CHICKPEA CURRY (page 68)	TUNA LAYERED LASAGNE (page 54)	SWEDISH MEATBALLS (page 86)

Essential Equipment

If you're starting from scratch you'll probably have to beg or borrow most of your kitchen equipment, which means you won't be cooking with state-of-the-art pans and processors. But you don't actually need many gadgets and gizmos to rustle up any of the recipes in this book.

With just a few basics you can eat well and even impress your friends with more daring creations when you develop some culinary confidence. Here's a list of the equipment you'll need in order to avoid a bread and baked beans diet.

Utensils Measuring jug, two different-sized mixing bowls, wooden spoon, rolling pin, grater, spatula, chopping board, vegetable peeler, whisk, colander, sharp knives (one small for prepping veg and one large for chopping, slicing bread etc).

Pots and pans Large and small saucepan (with lids), large nonstick frying pan, steamer (very useful but a metal colander over a pan will work fine). A wok is also handy for quick stir-fries, but not essential.

Cookware Baking sheet, roasting tin, flameproof casserole dish, large rectangular ovenproof dish (for lasagnes, bakes etc), wire cooling rack, cake tins, muffin tin and pastry cutters (if you're a baker).

A blender or food processor is a luxury item that will prove useful if you find your cooking mojo. But don't worry if you can't get your hands on these pricier pieces of culinary kit – a relatively inexpensive hand blender will do the job for most soups and smoothies and your knife skills will be all the better for chopping everything by hand.

Five a day

It's common knowledge that we should all aim to eat at least five portions of fresh fruit and vegetables every day but it's easy to lose track, particularly when you're busy working and socializing, and grabbing food on the go. However, if you want to stay healthy, this is a quick and easy way to cram plenty of vitamins and minerals into your diet.

High five

1 Get in the habit of having fruit with breakfast and you've already earned one of your five before you leave the house – this could be chopped fruit on muesli or granola, a glass of fresh juice, or a banana on your cornflakes or porridge.

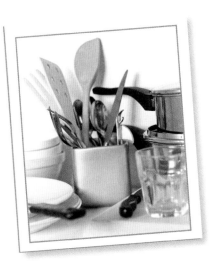

2 Steam vegetables as an accompaniment to dinner or have a side salad.

3 Switch your usual mid-morning bag of crisps for some chopped carrots and hummus.

4 Try ordering a fruit smoothie instead of that double-shot latte – you'll get the same buzz while upping your daily dose of fruit.

5 Tuck into a baked potato or toast piled high with baked beans – pulses count as one portion so there's no need to miss out on a lunchtime fave.

Healthy habits

It's easy to get into bad habits when you're responsible for all your own food shopping and meal prep. You might have the best intentions about staying hea... and eating a nutritious and balanced diet, but when you're dashing straight fro... lecture theatre to the pub, or you're craving a sugar hit to get you through a marathon essay-writing session, it's easy to fall off the wellbeing wagon and rea... for salty snacks, energy drinks and chocolate bars.

Sugar rush Sugar offers a short-term solution to lethargy but it won't keep you company for very long, as the initial buzz is swiftly followed by an energy lapse a... a craving for more sugary junk food. It's the added sugars in food and drink that... the real enemy, especially if the food doesn't have any other redeeming nutrition... features. Food labelling is becoming more transparent, so always check the label... see just how much sugar the product contains and to give yourself a reality check... and a nudge to choose a healthier alternative.

Fizzy drinks, processed snacks, some breakfast cereals and pasta sauces are all major culprits, but making simple changes like switching to porridge for breakfast... making your own sauce and cutting out the unnecessary biscuits and chocolate ba... can all make a big difference. And do you really need two or three spoons of sugar i... your morning coffee? Think of added sugar as empty calories – something your bod... doesn't need and something you can easily train it not to crave.

Call time on drinking A healthy lifestyle doesn't mean you have to treat your body like a temple 24/7. It's all about balance and making sensible choices most of the time. As long as you're aware of what you should be eating and drinking, the odd splurge or treat isn't the end of the world.

The same is true for drinking – student life wouldn't quite be the same if you sipped on a sparkling water in the union bar or slurped on smoothies at parties and club nights. But it's important to know your limitations and be aware of the number of units you're drinking. They can quickly add up, even during the more innocuous evenings in the pub. So, if you're out a few times a week, you're likely to be drinking far more than the recommended government guidelines, which are 2-3 units per day for women and 3-4 units per day for men.

Know your units

Women (2-3 units) a day
  1 pint average strength (4%) beer or cider
  Medium (175ml) glass of wine
  2-3 shots (25ml) of spirits

Men (3-4 units) a day
  1½ pints average strength (4%) beer or cider
  Large (250ml) glass of wine
  3-4 shots (25ml) of spirits

Mood boosters

Leaving home for the first time is a major life event and while it signals a huge leap in your independence, it can also have a big impact on your emotional state. It's normal to feel homesick and, as previously mentioned, it's important to take care of yourself by eating well, exercising and not overindulging on the alcohol front. As you settle into your course you'll also be putting a lot of pressure on your brain, which makes it even more important to boost your body with bundles of vitamin-rich foods. If you're having a bad day, feeling tired and finding it difficult to concentrate, there are a few foods that can help lift you up and give you a boost. Here are five to get you started:

Water We should drink about 1.5–2 litres of fluid a day and the more of that amount that's made up of water, the better. A small drop in the amount of fluid you drink can very quickly affect your mood and you'll begin to get dehydrated, have a headache and feel tired.

Dark chocolate Yes, it does contain sugar, but dark chocolate also releases endorphins (happy chemicals) in your brain. Of course, everything in moderation so stick to a couple of squares – just enough to put a smile on your face.

Oily fish Salmon, sardines, mackerel and tuna all contain omega-3, which is an important nutrient that can help enhance your mood by calming you down if you feel stressed.

Green tea This should be your hot beverage of choice when you're revising for exams – the thiamine in green tea can help you concentrate.

Carbohydrates These are a vital part of a balanced diet and if you cut out the carbs you might not feel on top form. Carbs help your brain to produce serotonin and a regular intake of slow-release, wholegrain carbohydrates will help to keep you focused and full of energy.

Prep & cook times

You'll need to have some idea how long it will be until dinner's on the table, so each recipe is marked with a handy symbol:

Timing = 20 minutes and under

Timing = 20–40 minutes

Timing = 40+ minutes

Brekky and Lunchbox

berry, honey &
yogurt pots

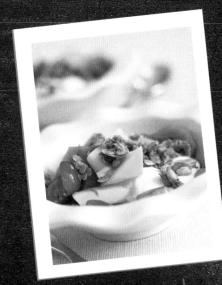

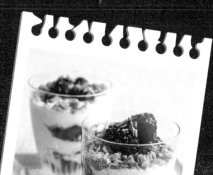

maple-glazed granola
with fruit

breakfast smoothie

banana & peanut butter smoothie

mango & orange smoothie

avocado & banana smoothie

gingered apple & carrot juice

watermelon cooler

cucumber lassi

berry, honey & yogurt pots

blueberry, oat & honey crumble

apple, yogurt museli

maple-glazed granola with fruit

mixed grain porridge

banana & sultana drop scones

porridge with prune compote

wholemeal blueberry pancakes with lemon curd yogurt

on-the-go granola breakfast bars

seeded spelt soda bread

falafel pitta pockets

falafels with beetroot salad & mint yogurt

brown rice salad with peanuts & raisins

pork & apple balls

sweet potato & bean 'steamed buns'

mushroom & rocket seeded wrap with feta & garlic dressing

blackened tofu wraps

breakfast smoothie

 Cost £

 Timing

 Serves 2-3

what You need

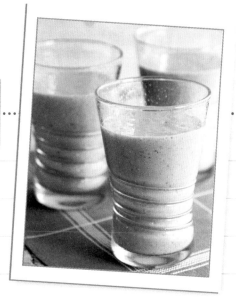

- 1 tablespoon pomegranate juice
- 1 small ripe banana, peeled and sliced
- 300 ml (½ pint) soya milk
- 1 tablespoon almonds
- 1 tablespoon rolled oats
- ½ teaspoon clear honey
- 1½ teaspoons ground linseeds
- 2 tablespoons natural yogurt

what You do

1. Place all the ingredients in a blender or food processor and blend until smooth and creamy.
2. Pour into 2-3 glasses and serve immediately.

TIPS Wake up and rehydrate Keep a large glass of water by your bed and drink it as soon as you wake up in the morning. This will help your body to rehydrate while you're getting ready for the day.

banana & peanut butter

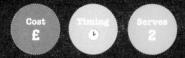

Cost £

Timing

Serves 2

what you need

- 1 ripe banana
- 300 ml (½ pint) semi-skimmed milk
- 1 tablespoon smooth peanut butter or 2 teaspoons tahini

what you do

1. Peel and slice the banana, put it in a freezer-proof container and freeze for at least 2 hours or overnight.
2. Put the frozen banana, the milk and peanut butter or tahini in a blender or food processor and blend until smooth.
3. Pour into 2 glasses and serve immediately.

NUTRITIONAL TIP

Tahini is a delicious paste made from crushed sesame seeds. Weight for weight, sesame seeds contain ten times more calcium than milk. This smoothie is an excellent source of vitamins C, B₁, B₂, B₆ and B₁₂, folic acid, niacin, calcium, copper, potassium, zinc, magnesium and phosphorus.

mango & orange smoothie

Cost
£

Timing

Serves
2

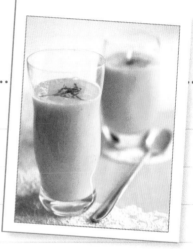

what you need

- 1 ripe mango, peeled, stoned and chopped, or 150 g (5 oz) frozen mango chunks
- 150 ml (¼ pint) natural soya yogurt
- 150 ml (¼ pint) orange juice
- finely grated rind and juice of 1 lime
- 2 teaspoons agave nectar, or to taste

what you do

1. Blend together the mango, yogurt, orange juice, lime rind and juice and agave nectar in a blender or food processor until smooth.
2. Pour into 2 glasses and serve immediately.

Variation
For mango lassi, cut the flesh of 1 ripe mango into cubes and add it to a blender or food processor with 150 ml (¼ pint) natural yogurt and the same amount of ice-cold water, 1 tablespoon rosewater and ¼ teaspoon ground cardamom. Blend briefly, then serve immediately.

avocado & banana smoothie

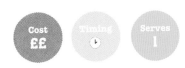

Cost
££

Timing

Serves
1

what you do

1. Peel the avocado, remove the stone and roughly chop the flesh. Peel and slice the banana.
2. Place the avocado, banana and milk in a blender or food processor and blend together until smooth.
3. Pour into a glass, add a couple of ice cubes and serve immediately.

what you need

- 1 small ripe avocado
- 1 small ripe banana
- 250 ml (8 fl oz) skimmed milk

HEALTHY TIP

In the tropics, avocados are often called poor man's butter because of their creamy texture and high fat content. Unlike butter, though, most of the fat is monounsaturated — the sort that helps lower levels of the 'bad' cholesterol (or low-density lipoproteins) while raising levels of the 'good' cholesterol (or high-density lipoproteins). Just one avocado provides around half the recommended daily intake of vitamin B6. This smoothie is an excellent source of vitamins C, E, B1, B2, B6 and B12, as well as folic acid, calcium, potassium, copper, zinc, magnesium and phosphorus.

gingered apple & carrot juice

what you need

Cost £   **Timing** ⏱   **Serves** 2

- 375 g (12 oz) carrots, peeled and cut into chunks
- 3 dessert apples, cored and cut into chunks
- 2.5 cm (1 inch) piece of fresh root ginger, peeled

what you do

1. Feed the carrot and apple chunks through a juicer with the ginger.
2. Pour the juice into 2 glasses and serve immediately.

watermelon cooler

Cost £   **Timing** ⏱   **Serves** 2

what you do

1. Skin and deseed the watermelon and chop the flesh into cubes. Hull the strawberries. Freeze the melon and strawberries until solid.
2. Put the frozen melon and strawberries into a blender or food processor, add the water and mint or tarragon and blend until smooth.
3. Pour the mixture into 2 glasses, garnish with mint or tarragon leaves, if liked, and serve immediately.

what you need

- 100 g (3½ oz) watermelon
- 100 g (3½ oz) strawberries
- 100 ml (3½ fl oz) water
- small handful of mint or tarragon leaves, plus extra to serve (optional)

cucumber lassi

what you need

- 150 g (5 oz) cucumber
- 150 ml (¼ pint) natural yogurt
- 100 ml (3⅓ fl oz) ice-cold water
- handful of mint
- ½ teaspoon ground cumin
- squeeze of lemon juice

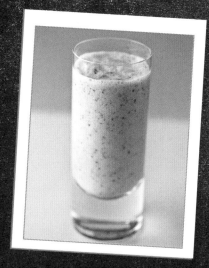

HEALTHY TIP

Smoothie does it.
If your fruit bowl is looking a little sad, with a couple of lonely items fast approaching over-ripeness, wash, peel, slice and blitz them up in a food processor or blender into a liquid vitamin boost. Add a dash of orange juice or other fruit juice if you need to boost the volume.

what you do

1. Peel and roughly chop the cucumber. Place in a blender or food processor with the yogurt and iced water.
2. Pull the mint leaves off their stalks, reserving a few for garnish. Chop the remainder roughly and put them into the blender. Add the cumin and lemon juice and blend briefly until smooth.
3. Pour the smoothie into a glass, garnish with mint leaves, if liked, and serve immediately.

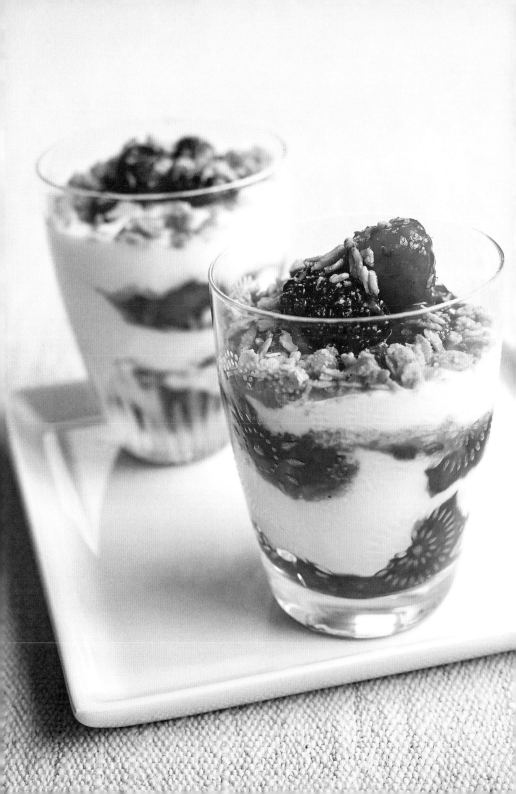

berry, honey & yogurt pots

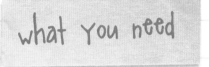

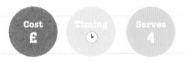

Cost
£

Timing

Serves
4

- 400 g (13 oz) frozen mixed berries, defrosted
- juice of 1 orange
- 6 tablespoons clear honey
- 400 ml (14 fl oz) vanilla yogurt
- 50 g (2 oz) granola

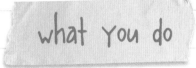

1. Whizz half of the berries with the orange juice and honey in a blender or food processor until fairly smooth.
2. Transfer to a bowl and stir in the remaining berries.
3. Divide one-third of the berry mixture between 4 glasses or small bowls. Top with half of the yogurt.
4. Layer with half of the remaining berry mixture and top with the remaining yogurt.
5. Top with the remaining berry mixture, then sprinkle over the granola just before serving.

blueberry, oat & honey crumble

Cost
£

Timing

Serves
1

what you do

1. Put the butter in a 200 ml (7 fl oz) microwave-proof mug and microwave on full power for 30 seconds or until melted.
2. Stir in the oats, sugar, honey and cinnamon and microwave on full power for 1 minute.
3. Mix well, then stir in the blueberries and microwave on full power for a further 1 minute until the blueberry juices start to run. Serve with Greek yogurt.

what you need

- 1 tablespoon unsalted butter
- 50 g (2 oz) rolled oats
- 1 tablespoon soft light brown sugar
- 2 teaspoons clear honey
- generous pinch of ground cinnamon
- 50 g (2 oz) blueberries
- 0%-fat Greek yogurt, to serve

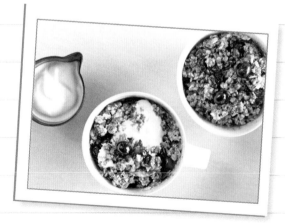

apple & yogurt muesli

Cost
££

Timing

Serves
2

what you need

- 75 g (3 oz) fruit and nut muesli, preferably no-added-sugar
- 1 dessert apple, such as Granny Smith, peeled, cored and coarsely grated
- 200 ml (7 fl oz) chilled apple juice
- 125 ml (4 fl oz) 0%-fat Greek yogurt with honey

To serve
- linseeds (optional)
- clear honey (optional)

what you do

1. Put the muesli in a bowl and mix with the grated apple. Pour over the apple juice, stir well to combine and leave to soak for 5–6 minutes.
2. Divide the soaked muesli between 2 serving bowls and spoon the yogurt on top.
3. Scatter over the linseeds, if using, and serve with a drizzle of honey, if liked.

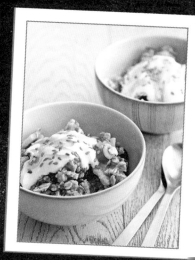

maple-glazed granola with fruit

what you need

Cost
££

Serves
6

- 2 tablespoons olive oil
- 2 tablespoons maple syrup
- 40 g (1½ oz) flaked almonds
- 40 g (1½ oz) pine nuts
- 25 g (1 oz) sunflower seeds
- 25 g (1 oz) porridge oats
- 375 ml (13 fl oz) natural yogurt

Fruit salad
- 1 ripe mango, peeled, stoned and sliced
- 2 kiwifruit, peeled and sliced
- small bunch of red seedless grapes, halved
- finely grated rind and juice of 1 lime

what you do

1. Heat the oil in an ovenproof frying pan, then add the maple syrup, nuts, seeds and oats and toss together.
2. Transfer the pan to a preheated oven, 180°C (350°F), Gas Mark 4, and cook for 5–8 minutes, stirring once and moving the brown edges to the centre, until the granola mixture is evenly toasted.
3. Leave the mixture to cool, then pack it into a storage jar, seal, label and consume within 10 days.

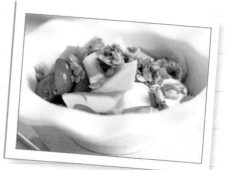

4. Make the fruit salad. Mix the fruits with the lime rind and juice, spoon the mixture into bowls and top with spoonfuls of natural yogurt and granola.

mixed grain porridge

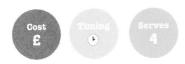

Cost
£

Timing

Serves
4

what you need

- 50 g (2 oz) buckwheat flakes
- 50 g (2 oz) quinoa flakes
- 50 g (2 oz) millet flakes
- 600 ml (1 pint) semi-skimmed milk
- 300 ml (½ pint) water
- 2 bananas, peeled

To serve
- 4 tablespoons 0%-fat Greek yogurt
- clear honey or maple syrup
- sprinkling of ground cinnamon

what you do

1. Put the grain flakes, milk and water into a saucepan and bring to the boil, then reduce the heat and cook for 4–5 minutes, stirring until thickened.
2. Mash 1 of the bananas and slice the other. Stir the mashed banana into the porridge, then spoon into bowls and top with spoonfuls of yogurt, the sliced banana, a drizzle of honey or maple syrup and a sprinkling of cinnamon. Serve immediately.

NUTRITIONAL TIP

Use unsweetened soya milk instead of dairy milk, if you prefer. If you use soya yogurt rather than Greek yogurt, this dish will be suitable for a dairy-free or vegan diet.

banana & sultana drop scones

Cost
£

Timing

Serves
10

what you need

- 125 g (4 oz) self-raising flour
- 2 tablespoons caster sugar
- ½ teaspoon baking powder
- 1 small ripe banana, about 125 g (4 oz) with skin on, peeled and roughly mashed
- 1 egg, beaten
- 150 ml (¼ pint) milk
- 50 g (2 oz) sultanas
- vegetable oil, for greasing
- butter, clear honey, or golden or maple syrup, to serve

Variation
For summer berry drop scones, prepare the recipe as above, but stir in 125 g (4 oz) mixed fresh blueberries and raspberries instead of the sultanas.

what you do

1. Put the flour, sugar and baking powder in a mixing bowl. Add the mashed banana with the egg. Gradually whisk in the milk with a fork until the mixture resembles a smooth thick batter. Stir in the sultanas.
2. Pour a little oil on to a piece of folded kitchen paper and use to grease a griddle or heavy-based nonstick frying pan. Heat the pan, then drop heaped dessertspoonfuls of the mixture (in batches), well spaced apart, on to the pan. Cook for 2 minutes until bubbles appear on the top and the undersides are golden. Turn over and cook for a further 1–2 minutes until the second side is done.
3. Serve warm, topped with 1 teaspoon butter, honey, or golden or maple syrup per scone. These are best eaten on the day they are made.

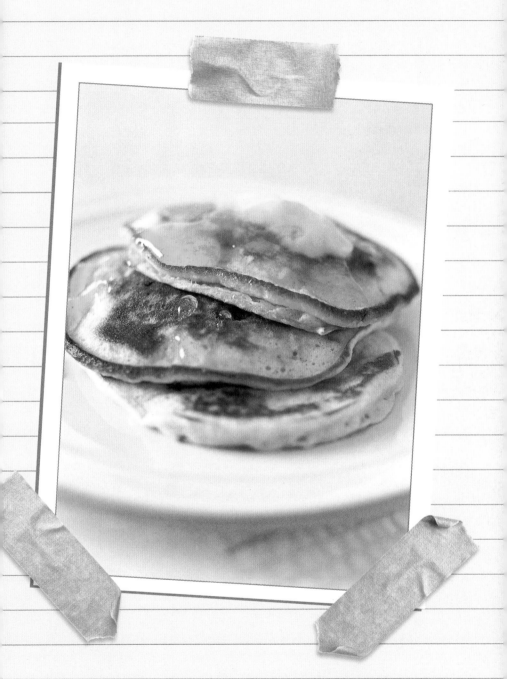

porridge with prune compote

what you need

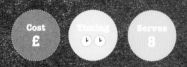

Cost £ · **Timing** · **Serves** 8

- 1 litre (1¾ pints) skimmed or semi-skimmed milk
- 500 ml (17 fl oz) water
- 1 teaspoon vanilla extract
- pinch of ground cinnamon
- pinch of salt
- 200 g (7 oz) porridge oats
- 3 tablespoons flaked almonds, toasted

Compote
- 250 g (8 oz) ready-to-eat pitted dried Agen prunes
- 125 ml (4 fl oz) apple juice
- 1 small cinnamon stick
- 1 whole clove
- 1 tablespoon clear honey
- 1 unpeeled orange quarter

what you do

1. Place all the compote ingredients in a small saucepan over a medium heat. Simmer gently for 10–12 minutes or until softened and slightly sticky. Leave to cool. (The compote can be prepared in advance and chilled. Remember to remove the cinnamon stick and clove before serving.)
2. Put the milk, water, vanilla extract, cinnamon and salt in a large saucepan over a medium heat and bring slowly to the boil. Stir in the oats, then reduce the heat and simmer gently, stirring occasionally, for 8–10 minutes until creamy and tender.
3. Spoon the porridge into bowls, scatter with the almonds and serve with the prune compote.

Variation

For sweet quinoa porridge with banana and dates, put 250 g (8 oz) quinoa in a saucepan with the milk, 1 tablespoon agave nectar or clear honey and 2–3 cardamom pods, crushed. Simmer gently for 12–15 minutes or until the quinoa is cooked and the desired consistency is reached. Discard the cardamom pods. Serve the porridge in bowls topped with a dollop of natural yogurt, 100 g (3½ oz) chopped pitted dates and sliced banana.

wholemeal blueberry pancakes with lemon curd yogurt

Cost	Timing	Serves
££	▸ ▸	4

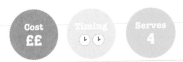

what You need

- 150 g (5 oz) wholemeal plain flour
- 50 g (2 oz) plain flour
- 1 teaspoon baking powder
- 300 ml (½ pint) milk
- 1 egg, beaten
- 2 tablespoons clear honey, plus extra for drizzling
- 175 g (6 oz) blueberries
- 25 g (1 oz) coconut oil
- 1 tablespoon lemon curd
- 125 ml (4 fl oz) natural yogurt

what You do

1. Sift the flours and baking powder into a large bowl, then make a well in the centre. Mix together the milk, egg and honey in a jug, then pour into the dry ingredients and whisk until mixed. Stir in 150 g (5 oz) of the blueberries.

2. Heat the coconut oil in a large frying pan, then drop 2 tablespoons of the batter into the pan for each pancake to form 4 and cook for 4–5 minutes until golden, then turn over and cook for a further 2–3 minutes. Remove from the pan and keep warm. Repeat with the remaining batter to make about 12.

3. Mix together the lemon curd and yogurt in a small bowl. Serve the warm pancakes with dollops of the lemon yogurt, sprinkled with the remaining blueberries and drizzled with honey.

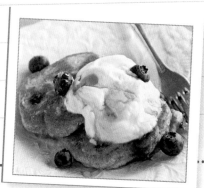

on-the-go granola breakfast bars

Cost ££   **Timing**   **Serves** 9

- 75 g (3 oz) butter, plus extra for greasing
- 75 ml (3 fl oz) clear honey
- ½ teaspoon ground cinnamon
- 100 g (3½ oz) ready-to-eat dried apricots, roughly chopped
- 50 g (2 oz) ready-to-eat dried papaya or mango, roughly chopped

- 50 g (2 oz) raisins
- 4 tablespoons mixed seeds, such as pumpkin, sesame and sunflower
- 50 g (2 oz) pecan nuts, roughly broken
- 150 g (5 oz) porridge oats

what you do

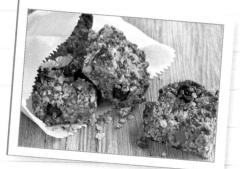

1. Grease a shallow 20 cm (8 inch) square tin.
2. Place the butter and honey in a saucepan and bring gently to the boil, stirring continuously, until the mixture bubbles. Add the cinnamon, dried fruit, seeds and nuts, then stir and heat for 1 minute.
3. Remove from the heat and add the oats. Stir well, then transfer to the prepared tin and press down well. Bake in a preheated oven, 190°C (375°F), Gas Mark 5, for 15 minutes until the top is just beginning to brown.
4. Leave to cool in the tin, then cut into 9 squares or bars to serve. Store in an airtight tin for up to 2 days.

seeded spelt soda bread

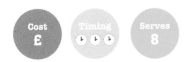

Cost
£

Timing

Serves
8

what you need

- vegetable oil, for greasing
- 250 g (8 oz) spelt flour, plus extra for dusting
- 100 g (3½ oz) rye flour
- 2 teaspoons baking powder
- 1 teaspoon salt
- 40 g (1½ oz) pumpkin seeds
- 40 g (1½ oz) sunflower seeds
- 284 ml (9½ fl oz) carton buttermilk
- 100 ml (3½ fl oz) semi-skimmed milk

STUDENT TIP

Breadcrumbs.

When you get to the last slice of bread, don't throw it away if it's a bit dry — blitz it in a blender and keep the breadcrumbs in an airtight container in the freezer. They're great for pie and bake toppings.

what you do

1. Grease a loaf tin with a capacity of at least 750 ml (1¼ pints). If you don't have a loaf tin, grease a baking sheet.
2. Sift the flours and baking powder into a bowl. Tip in the grain left in the sieve and stir in the salt and seeds. Add the buttermilk and milk and mix with a round-bladed knife to form a soft dough.
3. Turn out on to a lightly floured surface and shape into an oblong. Turn into the prepared tin or neaten the shape and place on the baking sheet. Bake in a preheated oven, 200°C (400°F), Gas Mark 6, for 20 minutes.
4. Reduce the oven temperature to 160°C (325°F), Gas Mark 3, and bake for a further 15 minutes. Turn out of the tin (if using) and return to the oven shelf for a further 10 minutes baking. Leave to cool completely on a wire rack. Serve in slices. This is best eaten on the day it is made.

falafel pitta pockets

what You need

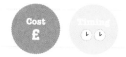

Cost £ · **Timing** · **Serves** 4

- 250 g (8 oz) dried chickpeas
- 1 small onion, finely chopped
- 2 garlic cloves, crushed
- ½ bunch of parsley
- ½ bunch of fresh coriander
- 2 teaspoons ground coriander
- ½ teaspoon baking powder
- 2 tablespoons vegetable oil
- 4 wholemeal pitta breads
- handful of salad leaves
- 2 tomatoes, diced
- 4 tablespoons 0%-fat Greek yogurt
- salt and pepper

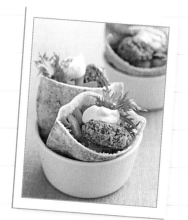

what You do

1. Put the chickpeas in a bowl, add cold water to cover by a generous 10 cm (4 inches) and leave to soak overnight.
2. Drain the chickpeas, transfer to a blender or food processor and process until coarsely ground. Add the onion, garlic, fresh herbs, ground coriander and baking powder. Season with salt and pepper and process until really smooth. Using wet hands, shape the mixture into 16 small patties.
3. Heat the oil in a large frying pan over a medium-high heat, add the patties, in batches, and fry for 3 minutes on each side or until golden and cooked through. Remove with a slotted spoon and drain on kitchen paper.
4. Split the pitta breads and fill with the falafel, salad leaves and diced tomatoes. Add a spoonful of the yogurt to each and serve immediately.

falafels with beetroot salad & mint yogurt

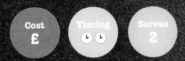

Cost
£

Timing
🌙 🌙

Serves
2

what you need

Falafels
- 400 g (13 oz) can chickpeas, rinsed and drained
- ¼ small red onion, roughly chopped
- 1 garlic clove, chopped
- ½ red chilli, deseeded
- 1 teaspoon ground cumin
- 1 teaspoon ground coriander
- handful of flat leaf parsley
- 2 tablespoons olive oil
- salt and pepper

Beetroot salad
- 1 carrot, coarsely grated
- 1 raw beetroot, coarsely grated
- 50 g (2 oz) baby spinach leaves
- 1 tablespoon lemon juice
- 2 tablespoons olive oil
-

Mint yogurt
- 150 ml (¼ pint) 0%-fat Greek yogurt
- 1 tablespoon chopped mint leaves
- ½ garlic clove, crushed

what you do

1. To make the falafels, place the chickpeas, onion, garlic, chilli, cumin, coriander and parsley in a blender or food processor. Season with salt and pepper, then process to make a coarse paste. Shape the mixture into 8 patties and set aside.

2. To make the salad, place the carrot, beetroot and spinach in a bowl. Season with salt and pepper, add the lemon juice and oil and stir well.

3. To make the mint yogurt, mix all the ingredients together in a small bowl and season with a little salt.

4. Heat the oil in a frying pan, add the falafels and fry for 4–5 minutes on each side until golden. Serve with the beetroot salad and mint yogurt.

brown rice salad with peanuts & raisins

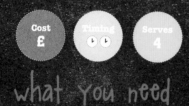

Cost £

Timing

Serves 4

what you need

- 200 g (7 oz) easy-cook brown rice
- bunch of spring onions, roughly chopped
- 125 g (4 oz) raisins
- 1 red pepper, cored, deseeded and sliced
- 75 g (3 oz) roasted peanuts
- 2 tablespoons dark soy sauce
- 1 tablespoon sesame oil
- salt

what you do

1. Cook the rice in a saucepan of lightly salted boiling water for 15–18 minutes until tender.
2. Meanwhile, place the spring onions, raisins, red pepper and peanuts in a large bowl and toss with the soy sauce and oil until well coated.
3. Once the rice is cooked, drain it in a sieve and rinse with cold water until cold. Once cold and drained, add to the other ingredients and toss well to coat and mix.
4. Turn into a serving bowl and serve, or place in a lunch box with slices of cheese or meat to serve alongside, if liked.

HEALTHY TIP

Go nuts for nuts.
The ultimate healthy snack but nuts can be quite pricey so buy a huge pack and divide it into smaller portions and you'll save money. Go for unsalted/unflavoured (natural) nuts and don't forget seeds (such as sunflower, pumpkin and linseeds) — a healthy snack and great for sprinkling.

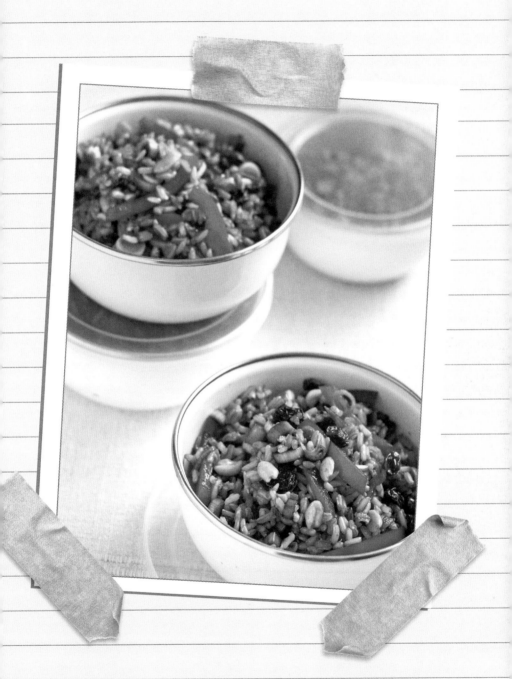

pork & apple balls

Cost
££

Timing

Serves
9

- 1 small dessert apple, such as Cox's, cored and grated (with skin on)
- 1 small onion, grated
- 250 g (8 oz) minced pork
- 50 g (2 oz) wholemeal breadcrumbs
- 3 tablespoons vegetable oil

To serve
- tomato chutney
- cherry tomatoes

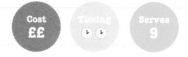

what you do

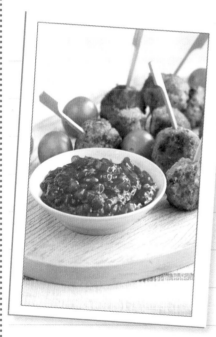

1. Place the apple and onion in a bowl with the minced pork and, using a fork, mash all the ingredients together well. Shape into 16 rough balls. Place the breadcrumbs on a plate and roll the balls in the breadcrumbs to lightly coat all over.
2. Heat the oil in a large, heavy-based frying pan and cook the pork balls over a medium-high heat for 8–10 minutes, turning frequently, until cooked through. Drain on kitchen paper.
3. Serve warm with tomato chutney and cherry tomatoes, and provide bamboo paddle skewers or forks for dipping the balls in the chutney.

sweet potato & bean 'steamed buns'

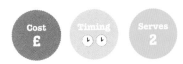

Cost
£

Timing

Serves
2

what you need

- 100 g (3½ oz) courgette, coarsely grated
- 1 teaspoon caster sugar
- 3 teaspoons rice vinegar
- 300 g (10 oz) sweet potatoes, scrubbed
- 100 g (3½ oz) French beans, trimmed and cut into 2.5 cm (1 inch) lengths
- 50 ml (2 fl oz) hoisin sauce
- 4 spring onions, thinly sliced
- 4 tablespoons chopped fresh coriander
- 2 wholemeal or white pitta breads

what you do

1. Mix the grated courgette with the sugar and 2 teaspoons of the vinegar in a small bowl and leave to stand while preparing the filling.
2. Thinly slice the sweet potatoes and cook in a saucepan of boiling water for 8–10 minutes until just tender. Add the beans and cook for a further 2 minutes to soften. Drain.
3. Add the hoisin sauce and the remaining vinegar to the saucepan. Tip in the drained vegetables, spring onions and coriander and mix well.
4. Wrap the pitta breads in clingfilm and microwave on full power for 1–2 minutes until soft.
5. Split the pittas and fill with the sweet potato mixture. Spoon the courgette mixture on top, then serve.

mushroom & rocket seeded wrap with feta & garlic dressing

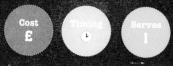

Cost £

Timing

Serves 1

what you need

- 40 g (1½ oz) feta cheese
- 50 ml (2 fl oz) 0%-fat Greek yogurt
- 1 tablespoon olive oil
- 200 g (7 oz) mushrooms, trimmed and thinly sliced
- ½ teaspoon garam masala
- 1 seeded wrap
- 25 g (1 oz) sprouting beans
- small handful of rocket, about 15 g (½ oz)
- 1 teaspoon clear honey
- salt and pepper

what you do

1. Crumble the feta into a small bowl and stir in the yogurt. Season with plenty of pepper and beat well with a fork.
2. Heat the olive oil in a small frying pan and fry the mushrooms for about 5 minutes until beginning to colour and the juices have evaporated. Stir in the garam masala and a pinch of salt and cook for a further 2 minutes.
3. Lightly grill the wrap under a preheated hot grill until warmed through. Spread with the feta mixture and tip the mushrooms on top. Scatter with the beans and rocket and drizzle with the honey. Roll up loosely to serve.

blackened tofu wraps

Cost	Timing	Serves
££	⏱	2

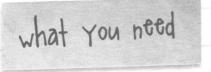

what you need

- 200 g (7 oz) firm tofu
- 1 tablespoon dark muscovado sugar
- 1 teaspoon pepper
- 1 teaspoon five-spice powder
- ½ teaspoon ground ginger
- 1 garlic clove, crushed
- 2 seeded wraps
- 2 tablespoons sesame oil
- 50 g (2 oz) mixed salad leaves
- 1 carrot, grated
- ½ bunch of spring onions, thinly sliced
- 1 tablespoon clear honey
- squeeze of lime or lemon juice
- salt

what you do

1. Thoroughly drain the tofu between several sheets of kitchen paper. Cut into thin slices. Mix together the sugar, pepper, five-spice powder, ginger and a little salt. Spread the garlic over the tofu, then dust on both sides with the spice mixture.
2. Warm the wraps in a frying pan or under a preheated hot grill.
3. Heat 1 tablespoon of the oil in a frying pan and fry the tofu slices for 1-2 minutes on each side until deep golden.
4. Scatter the salad leaves, carrot and spring onions over the warm wraps, then place the tofu slices on top, placing them over the length of the wraps.
5. Add the remaining oil, the honey and lime or lemon juice to the pan and stir to mix. Drizzle over the wraps, roll and then serve warm or cold.

Healthy and Hearty

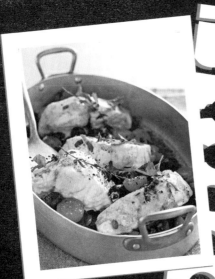

baked cod with
tomatoes & olives

hearty minestrone

summer vegetable soup

red pepper & courgette soup

beef & barley brö

butternut & rosemary soup

squash, kale & mixed bean soup

sweet potato & cabbage soup

aubergine cannelloni

spaghetti carbonara

linguine with shredded ham
& eggs

bolognese sauce

tuna layered lasagne

tuna & olive pasta

salmon with green vegetables

tuna & jalapeño baked potatoes

macaroni cheese surprise

ranch-style eggs ....

spinach & butternut lasagne ....

spinach & potato tortilla ....

butternut squash & ricotta frittata ....

kedgeree-style rice with spinach ....

barley & ginger risotto with butternut squash ....

lemon & herb risotto ....

mixed bean & tomato chilli ....

cauliflower & chickpea curry ....

vegetable curry with rice ....

vegetable, fruit & nut biryani ....

baked sweet potatoes ....

caribbean chicken with rice & peas ....

chicken & spinach stew ....

chicken jalfrezi ....

chicken shawarma ....

jambalaya with chorizo & peppers ....

chicken burgers with tomato salsa ....

chicken fajitas with no-chilli salsa ....

pot roast chicken ....

roast lemony chicken with courgettes ....

warm chicken, med veg & bulgar wheat salad ....

oven-baked turkey & gruyére burgers ....

swedish meatballs ....

steak meatloaf ....

roast pork loin with creamy cabbage & leeks ....

garlicky pork with warm butter bean salad ....

one-pan spiced pork ....

spicy sausage bake ....

cheesy pork with parsnip purée ....

chorizo, ham & eggs ....

butter bean & chorizo stew ....

west indian beef & bean stew ....

beef, pumpkin & prune stew ....

baked cod with tomatoes & olives ....

haddock with poached eggs ....

smoked mackerel kedgeree ....

quick tuna fishcakes ....

red salmon & roasted vegetables ....

hearty minestrone

what you need

3 carrots, roughly chopped
1 red onion, roughly chopped
3 celery sticks, roughly chopped
2 tablespoons olive oil
2 garlic cloves, crushed
200 g (7 oz) potatoes, peeled and
cut into 1 cm (½ inch) dice
4 tablespoons tomato purée
1.5 litres (2½ pints) Vegetable
Stock (see page 164)
400 g (13 oz) can chopped
tomatoes
150 g (5 oz) short-shaped soup
pasta
400 g (13 oz) can cannellini
beans, rinsed and drained
100 g (3½ oz) baby spinach
salt and pepper
crusty bread, to serve

Cost	Timing	Serves
£	⏱ ⏱	4

what you do

1. Whizz the carrots, onion and celery in a blender or food processor until finely chopped.
2. Heat the oil in a large saucepan, add the chopped vegetables, garlic, potatoes, tomato purée, stock, tomatoes and pasta. Bring to the boil, then reduce the heat and simmer, covered, for 12–15 minutes, stirring occasionally.
3. Tip in the cannellini beans and the spinach for the final 2 minutes of the cooking time.
4. Season to taste with salt and pepper and serve with crusty bread.

HEALTHY TIP

Wise up to water.

It really is the elixir of life so try to make sure you drink more aqua than alcohol. Keep a bottle in your bag and drink regularly throughout the day to keep your brain alert and lethargy at bay.

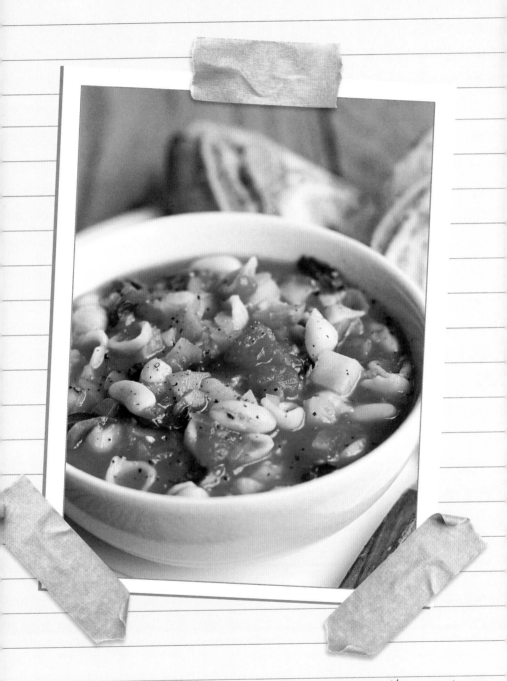

Healthy and Hearty **43**

summer vegetable soup

Cost
£

Timing
⏱ ⏱

Serves
4

what you need

- 1 teaspoon olive oil
- 1 leek, trimmed, cleaned and thinly sliced
- 1 large potato, peeled and chopped
- 900 ml (1½ pints) Vegetable Stock (see page 164)
- 450 g (14½ oz) prepared

mixed summer vegetables (such as peas, asparagus, broad beans and courgettes)
- 2 tablespoons chopped mint
- 2 tablespoons half-fat crème fraîche
- salt and pepper

what you do

1. Heat the oil in a medium saucepan and fry the leek for 3–4 minutes until softened. Add the potato and stock to the pan and cook for 10 minutes. Add the mixed summer vegetables and the mint, then bring to the boil. Reduce the heat and simmer, stirring occasionally, for 10 minutes.
2. Cool slightly, then transfer the soup to a blender or food processor and purée until smooth. Return the soup to the pan, add the crème fraîche and season to taste with salt and pepper. Heat through gently and serve.

Variation

For chunky summer vegetable soup with mixed herb gremolata, make up the soup as above but do not purée. Ladle the soup into bowls and serve topped with 2 tablespoons crème fraîche and gremolata, made by mixing together 2 tablespoons chopped basil, 2 tablespoons chopped parsley, the finely grated rind of 1 lemon and 1 finely chopped small garlic clove.

red pepper & courgette soup

what you do

1. Heat the oil in a large saucepan and gently fry the onions for 5 minutes or until softened and golden brown. Add the garlic and cook gently for 1 minute. Add the red peppers and half of the courgettes to the pan. Fry for 5–8 minutes or until softened and brown.
2. Add the stock to the pan, season to taste with salt and pepper and bring to the boil. Reduce the heat, cover the pan and simmer gently, stirring occasionally, for 20 minutes.
3. Allow the soup to cool slightly once the vegetables are tender, then purée in batches in a blender or food processor. Gently fry the remaining chopped courgettes for 5 minutes (you may need to add a little more oil to the pan).
4. Meanwhile, return the soup to the pan, reheat gently, then taste and adjust the seasoning if needed. Serve topped with the fried courgettes, yogurt or crème fraîche and chives.

what you need

- 2 tablespoons olive oil
- 2 onions, finely chopped
- 1 garlic clove, crushed
- 3 red peppers, cored, deseeded and roughly chopped
- 2 courgettes, roughly chopped
- 900 ml (1½ pints) Vegetable Stock (see page 164)
- salt and pepper

To serve
- low-fat natural yogurt or half-fat crème fraîche
- whole chives

Variation
For red pepper and carrot soup, make up the soup as above, adding 2 diced carrots instead of the courgettes, plus the red peppers, to the fried onion and garlic. Continue as above. Purée, reheat and serve topped with teaspoonfuls of garlic and herb soft cheese and some snipped chives.

beef & barley brö

- 25 g (1 oz) butter
- 250 g (8 oz) braising beef, fat trimmed away and meat cut into small cubes
- 1 large onion, finely chopped
- 200 g (7 oz) swede, diced
- 150 g (5 oz) carrot, diced

- 100 g (3½ oz) pearl barley
- 2 litres (3½ pints) beef stock
- 2 teaspoons dry English mustard (optional)
- salt and pepper
- chopped parsley, to garnish

what you do

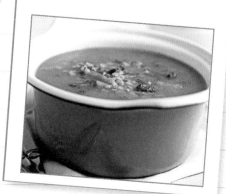

1. Melt the butter in a large saucepan, then add the beef and onion and fry for 5 minutes, stirring, until the beef is browned and the onion is just beginning to colour.

2. Stir in the diced vegetables, pearl barley, stock and mustard, if using. Season with salt and pepper and bring to the boil. Cover and simmer for 1¾ hours, stirring occasionally, until the meat and vegetables are very tender. Taste and adjust the seasoning if needed.

3. Ladle the soup into bowls and sprinkle with a little chopped parsley just before serving.

butternut
& rosemary soup

Cost
£

Timing

Serves
4

what you need

- 1 butternut squash, halved, deseeded and cut into small chunks
- few rosemary sprigs, plus extra leaves to garnish
- 150 g (5 oz) red lentils, rinsed and drained
- 1 onion, finely chopped
- 900 ml (1½ pints) Vegetable Stock (see page 164)
- salt and pepper

what you do

1. Place the squash pieces in a nonstick roasting tin. Sprinkle over the rosemary sprigs and season with salt and pepper. Roast in a preheated oven, 200°C (400°F), Gas Mark 6, for 45 minutes.
2. Meanwhile, put the lentils in a saucepan and cover with water, then bring to the boil and boil rapidly for 10 minutes. Drain, then return to a clean saucepan with the onion and stock and simmer for 5 minutes. Season with salt and pepper.
3. Remove the squash from the oven and scoop the flesh from the skin. Next, mash the flesh with a fork and add it to the soup, then simmer for 25 minutes, stirring occasionally, until the lentils are tender. Serve the soup scattered with extra rosemary.

squash, kale & mixed bean soup

Cost
£

Timing
● ● ●

Serves
6

- 1 tablespoon olive oil
- 1 onion, finely chopped
- 2 garlic cloves, finely chopped
- 1 teaspoon smoked paprika
- 500 g (1 lb) butternut squash, halved, deseeded, peeled and diced
- 2 small carrots, peeled and diced
- 500 g (1 lb) tomatoes, skinned (optional) and roughly chopped
- 400 g (13 oz) can mixed beans, rinsed and drained
- 900 ml (1½ pints) Vegetable Stock (see page 164)
- 150 ml (¼ pint) half-fat crème fraîche
- 100 g (3½ oz) kale, torn into bite-sized pieces
- salt and pepper
- crusty bread or warm garlic bread, to serve (optional)

what you do

1. Heat the oil in a saucepan over a medium-low heat, add the onion and fry gently for 5 minutes. Stir in the garlic and smoked paprika and cook briefly, then add the squash, carrots, tomatoes and mixed beans. Pour in the stock, season with salt and pepper and bring to the boil, stirring frequently. Reduce the heat, cover and simmer for 25 minutes, stirring occasionally, until the vegetables are cooked and tender.

2. Stir in the crème fraîche, then add the kale, pressing it just beneath the surface of the stock. Cover and cook for 5 minutes or until the kale has just wilted. Ladle the soup into bowls and serve with warm garlic bread, if liked.

Variation

For cheesy squash, pepper and mixed bean soup, make as above, replacing the carrots with 1 cored, deseeded and diced red pepper. Pour in the stock, then add 65 g (2¼ oz) Parmesan-style cheese rinds and season. Cover and simmer for 25 minutes. Stir in the crème fraîche but omit the kale. Discard the cheese rinds, ladle the soup into bowls and top with grated Parmesan-style cheese.

sweet potato & cabbage soup

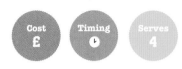

Cost £   **Timing** ⏱   **Serves** 4

what you do

what you need

- 2 onions, chopped
- 2 garlic cloves, sliced
- 4 lean back bacon rashers, chopped
- 500 g (1 lb) sweet potatoes, scrubbed or peeled and chopped
- 2 parsnips, chopped
- 1 teaspoon chopped thyme
- 900 ml (1½ pints) Vegetable Stock (see page 164)
- 1 baby Savoy cabbage, shredded
- Irish soda bread, to serve

what you do

1. Place the onions, garlic and bacon in a large saucepan and fry for 2–3 minutes. Add the sweet potatoes, parsnips, thyme and stock to the saucepan, then bring to the boil and simmer for 15 minutes, stirring occasionally.

2. Cool slightly, then transfer two-thirds of the soup to a blender or food processor and blend until smooth. Return to the pan, add the cabbage and simmer for 5–7 minutes until the cabbage is just cooked. Serve with Irish soda bread.

Variation

For squash and broccoli soup, follow the recipe above, replacing the sweet potatoes with 500 g (1 lb) peeled, deseeded and chopped butternut squash. After returning the blended soup to the pan, add 100 g (3½ oz) small broccoli florets. Cook as above, omitting the cabbage.

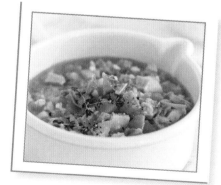

aubergine cannelloni

what you need

- 4 sheets of fresh or dried lasagne, each about 18 x 15 cm (7 x 6 inches)
- 2 medium aubergines, thinly sliced
- 4 tablespoons olive oil
- 1 teaspoon finely chopped thyme
- 250 g (8 oz) ricotta cheese
- 25 g (1 oz) basil leaves, torn into pieces
- 2 garlic cloves, crushed
- 1 quantity Fresh Tomato Sauce (see page 169)
- 100 g (3½ oz) fontina or Gruyère cheese, grated
- salt and pepper

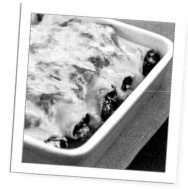

what you do

1. Bring a saucepan of lightly salted water to the boil. Add the lasagne sheets, return to the boil and cook, allowing 2 minutes for fresh and 8–10 minutes for dried. Drain the sheets and immerse in cold water.
2. Place the aubergine slices in a single layer on a foil-lined grill rack. (You may need to do this in 2 batches.) Mix together the oil, thyme and some salt and pepper and brush over the aubergines. Grill under a preheated medium-hot grill until lightly browned all over, turning once.
3. Beat the ricotta in a bowl with the basil, garlic and a little salt and pepper. Thoroughly drain the pasta sheets and lay them on the work surface. Cut each one in half. Spread the ricotta mixture over the lasagne sheets, right to the edges. Arrange the aubergine slices on top. Roll up each pasta sheet to enclose the filling inside.
4. Spread two-thirds of the tomato sauce in a shallow ovenproof dish and arrange the cannelloni on top. Spoon over the remaining tomato sauce and then sprinkle with the cheese. Bake in a preheated oven, 190°C (375°F), Gas Mark 5, for 20 minutes or until the cheese is golden.

spaghetti carbonara

- 4 egg yolks
- 2 eggs
- 150 ml (¼ pint) single cream
- 50 g (2 oz) Parmesan cheese, grated
- 2 tablespoons olive oil
- 100 g (3½ oz) pancetta or streaky bacon, thinly sliced
- 2 garlic cloves, crushed
- 400 g (13 oz) fresh spaghetti
- salt and pepper

what you do

1. Beat together the egg yolks, whole eggs, cream, Parmesan and plenty of pepper.
2. Heat the oil in a large frying pan and fry the pancetta or bacon for 3–4 minutes or until golden and turning crisp. Add the garlic and cook for a further 1 minute.
3. Meanwhile, bring a large saucepan of lightly salted water to the boil, add the spaghetti and cook for 2 minutes or until tender.
4. Drain the spaghetti and immediately tip it into the frying pan. Turn off the heat and stir in the egg mixture until the eggs are lightly cooked. (If the heat of the pasta doesn't quite cook the egg sauce, turn on the heat and cook gently and briefly, stirring.) Serve immediately.

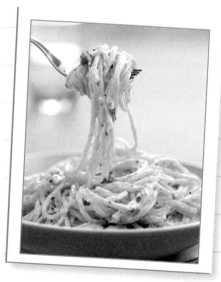

linguine with shredded ham & eggs

 Cost £

 Timing

 Serves 2

what you do

what you need

- 125 g (4 oz) dried linguine
- 3 tablespoons chopped flat leaf parsley
- 1 tablespoon wholegrain mustard
- 2 teaspoons lemon juice
- good pinch of caster sugar
- 3 tablespoons olive oil
- 100 g (3½ oz) ham
- 2 spring onions
- 2 eggs
- salt and pepper

1. Bring a large saucepan of lightly salted water to the boil to cook the pasta. Meanwhile, mix together the parsley, mustard, lemon juice, sugar, oil and a little salt and pepper. Roll up the ham and slice it as thinly as possible. Trim the spring onions, cut them lengthways into thin shreds, then cut into 5 cm (2 inch) lengths.

2. Put the eggs in a small saucepan and just cover with cold water. Bring to the boil and cook for 4 minutes.

3. Add the pasta to the large saucepan of boiling water, return to the boil and cook for 8–10 minutes or until just tender. Add the spring onions and cook for a further 30 seconds.

4. Drain the pasta and return to the pan. Stir in the ham and the mustard dressing and then pile on to serving plates. Shell and halve the eggs and serve on top.

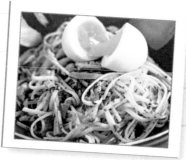

bolognese sauce

Cost
££

Timing
▶ ▶ ▶

Serves
4

what you need

- 15 g (½ oz) butter
- 3 tablespoons olive oil
- 1 large onion, finely chopped
- 1 celery stick, finely chopped
- 1 carrot, finely chopped
- 3 garlic cloves, crushed
- 500 g (1 lb) lean minced beef
- 150 ml (¼ pint) red wine
- 2 x 400 g (13 oz) cans chopped tomatoes
- 2 tablespoons sun-dried tomato paste
- 3 tablespoons chopped oregano
- 3 bay leaves
- salt and pepper
- grated Parmesan cheese, to serve (optional)

what you do

1. Melt the butter with the oil in a large, heavy-based saucepan and gently fry the onion for 5 minutes. Add the celery and carrot and fry gently for a further 2 minutes.

2. Stir in the garlic, then add the minced beef. Fry gently, breaking up the meat, until lightly browned.

3. Add the wine and let the mixture bubble until the wine reduces slightly. Stir in the chopped tomatoes, tomato paste, oregano and bay leaves and bring to the boil.

4. Reduce the heat and cook very gently, uncovered, for about 45 minutes, stirring occasionally, until the sauce is very thick and pulpy. Remove the bay leaves. Check and adjust the seasoning, then serve with grated Parmesan, if liked.

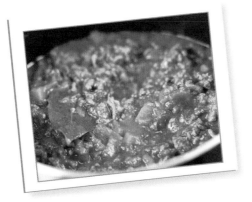

tuna layered lasagne

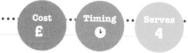

what you need

Cost £
Timing ⏱
Serves 4

- 8 dried lasagne sheets
- 1 tablespoon olive oil
- bunch of spring onions, sliced
- 2 courgettes, diced
- 500 g (1 lb) cherry tomatoes, quartered
- 2 x 200 g (7 oz) cans tuna in water, drained

- 65 g (2½ oz) rocket
- 4 teaspoons Pesto (see page 168)
- salt and pepper
- basil leaves, to garnish

what you do

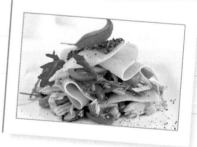

1. Cook the pasta sheets, in batches, in a large saucepan of lightly salted boiling water according to the packet instructions until al dente. Drain and return to the pan to keep warm.
2. Meanwhile, heat the oil in a frying pan over a medium heat, add the spring onions and courgettes and cook, stirring, for 3 minutes. Remove the pan from the heat, add the tomatoes, tuna and rocket and gently toss everything together.
3. Place a little of the tuna mixture on 4 serving plates and top each portion with a pasta sheet. Spoon over the remaining tuna mixture, then top with the remaining pasta sheets. Season with plenty of pepper and top each with a spoonful of pesto and some basil leaves before serving.

tuna & olive pasta

Cost
£

Timing

Serves
4

what you need

- 3 tablespoons olive or vegetable oil
- 1 red onion, sliced
- 2 garlic cloves, chopped
- 2 x 400 g (13 oz) cans chopped tomatoes
- ½ teaspoon dried chilli flakes (optional)
- 400 g (13 oz) pasta shapes, such as penne
- 185 g (6 ½ oz) can tuna in water or oil, drained and flaked
- 75 g (3 oz) pitted black or green olives, drained and roughly chopped
- salt

what you do

1. Heat the oil in a large frying pan or saucepan and cook the onion over a medium heat for 6-7 minutes until it begins to soften. Add the garlic and cook for a further 1 minute. Pour the chopped tomatoes into the pan with the chilli flakes, if using. Simmer gently for 8-10 minutes, stirring occasionally, until thickened slightly.
2. Meanwhile, bring a large saucepan of lightly salted water to the boil and cook the pasta for 10-12 minutes or according to the packet instructions until just tender. Drain and return to the pan. Stir the tomato sauce into the pasta with the tuna and olives and then heap into 4 dishes to serve.

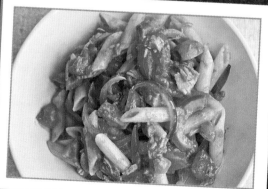

salmon with green vegetables

Cost
£££

Timing
▶ ▶

Serves
4

what you need

- 1 tablespoon olive oil
- 1 leek, trimmed, cleaned and thinly sliced
- 275 ml (9 fl oz) fish stock
- 200 ml (7 fl oz) half-fat crème fraîche
- 125 g (4 oz) frozen peas
- 125 g (4 oz) frozen edamame (soya) or broad beans
- 4 chunky skinless salmon fillets, about 150 g (5 oz) each
- 2 tablespoons snipped chives

To serve
- mashed potato
- pepper

what you do

1. Heat the oil in a large, heavy-based frying pan and cook the leek over a medium heat, stirring frequently, for 3 minutes until softened. Add the stock, then bring to the boil and continue boiling for 2 minutes until reduced a little. Add the crème fraîche and stir well to mix. Add the peas, edamame (soya) or broad beans and salmon and return to the boil.
2. Reduce the heat, cover and simmer for 10 minutes until the fish is opaque and cooked through and the peas and beans are piping hot.
3. Sprinkle over the chives and serve spooned over creamy mash with a good grinding of pepper.

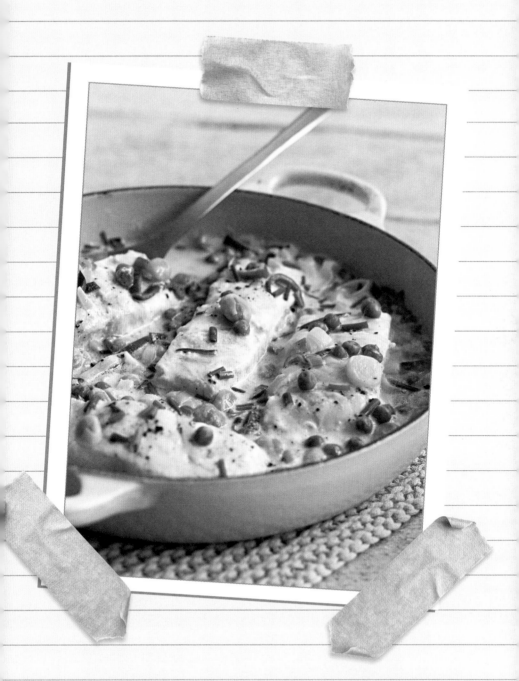

tuna & jalapeño baked potatoes

- 4 large baking potatoes
- 2 x 160 g (5½ oz) cans tuna in spring water, drained
- 2 tablespoons drained and chopped green jalapeño peppers in brine
- 2 spring onions, finely chopped
- 4 firm ripe tomatoes, deseeded and chopped
- 2 tablespoons snipped chives
- 3 tablespoons low-fat soured cream
- 100 g (3½ oz) reduced-fat extra mature Cheddar-style cheese, grated
- salt and pepper
- frisée salad, to serve

what you do

1. Prick the potatoes all over with the tip of a sharp knife and place directly in a preheated oven, 180°C (350°F), Gas Mark 4, for 1 hour or until crisp on the outside and the inside is tender. Leave until cool enough to handle.
2. Cut the potatoes in half and scoop the cooked flesh into a bowl. Place the empty potato skins, cut side up, on a baking sheet. Mix the tuna, jalapeño peppers, spring onions, tomatoes and chives into the potato in the bowl. Gently fold in the soured cream, then season to taste with salt and pepper.
3. Spoon the filling into the potato skins, sprinkle with the cheese and cook under a preheated medium-hot grill for 4–5 minutes or until hot and the cheese has melted. Serve immediately with a frisée salad.

macaroni cheese surprise

Cost
£

Timing
● ● ●

Serves
4

what you need

- 175 g (6 oz) wholemeal macaroni
- 2 carrots, cut into small, chunky batons
- 250 g (8 oz) broccoli florets
- 1 large leek, trimmed, cleaned and thickly sliced
- 50 g (2 oz) cornflour
- 600 ml (1 pint) skimmed milk
- 100 g (3½ oz) reduced-fat mature Cheddar-style cheese, grated
- 1 teaspoon mustard
- pinch of cayenne pepper, plus extra to garnish
- salt

what you do

1. Cook the macaroni in a large saucepan of lightly salted boiling water according to the packet instructions until just tender, then drain.
2. Meanwhile, lightly steam all the vegetables over a separate saucepan of boiling water so that they remain crunchy. Drain well.
3. Mix the cornflour and a little of the milk together in a saucepan. Blend to a smooth paste. Add the rest of the milk, then heat gently, whisking continuously until the sauce boils and thickens. Add three-quarters of the cheese, the mustard and cayenne pepper to taste.
4. Mix together the pasta, vegetables and sauce and spoon into an ovenproof dish. Scatter with the remaining cheese and sprinkle with a little cayenne pepper to garnish. Bake in a preheated oven, 200°C (400°F), Gas Mark 6, for about 25 minutes, until golden brown.

HEALTHY TIP

All pasta is naturally healthy — rich in carbohydrates and low in fat. Wholemeal pasta is made from the whole grain and contains more insoluble fibre than the white variety. This type of fibre helps to prevent constipation and other bowel problems.

ranch-style eggs

Cost £

Timing ◑ ◑

Serves 4

- 2 tablespoons olive oil
- 1 onion, thinly sliced
- 1 red chilli, deseeded and finely chopped
- 1 garlic clove, crushed
- 1 teaspoon ground cumin
- 1 teaspoon dried oregano
- 400 g (13 oz) can cherry tomatoes

- 200 g (7 oz) roasted red and yellow peppers in oil (from a jar), drained and roughly chopped
- 4 eggs
- salt and pepper
- 4 tablespoons finely chopped fresh coriander, to garnish

what You do

1. Heat the oil in a large frying pan and add the onion, chilli, garlic, cumin and oregano. Fry gently for about 5 minutes or until soft, then add the tomatoes and peppers and cook for a further 5 minutes. If the sauce looks dry, add a splash of water.
2. Season well with salt and pepper, then make 4 hollows in the mixture, break an egg into each and cover the pan. Cook for 5 minutes or until the eggs are just set.
3. Serve immediately, garnished with chopped coriander.

spinach & butternut lasagne

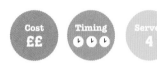

Cost **££**

Timing

Serves **4**

what you need

- 2 tablespoons olive oil
- 1 small butternut squash, about 700 g (1 lb 6 oz), deseeded, peeled and cut into small dice
- 1 teaspoon ground cumin
- ¼ teaspoon dried chilli flakes
- 400 g (13 oz) can chopped tomatoes
- 1 teaspoon caster sugar
- 200 g (7 oz) spinach
- 20 g (¾ oz) butter
- 2 tablespoons plain flour
- 300 ml (½ pint) semi-skimmed milk
- 100 g (3½ oz) mature Cheddar-type cheese, grated
- 100 g (3½ oz) dried lasagne sheets
- salt and pepper
- green salad, to serve

1. Heat the oil in a saucepan and gently fry the squash for 5 minutes, stirring. Add the cumin, chilli flakes, tomatoes and sugar and simmer gently, uncovered, for 20 minutes, stirring occasionally until the squash is tender. Stir in the spinach until wilted and season to taste with salt and pepper. Remove from the heat.

2. Melt the butter in a separate saucepan and stir in the flour, beating with a wooden spoon for 1 minute. Gradually stir in the milk and cook over a gentle heat, stirring continuously until thickened and smooth. Beat in half of the cheese and season to taste with salt and pepper. Remove from the heat.

3. Spread a quarter of the squash mixture into a shallow, ovenproof dish and cover with a layer of the lasagne sheets, breaking them to fit if necessary. Add another quarter of the squash mixture, spoon over about a third of the cheese sauce and cover with another layer of the lasagne sheets. Continue layering the ingredients in the same way, finishing with a layer of squash mixture topped with cheese sauce. Sprinkle with the remaining grated cheese.

4. Bake in a preheated oven, 190°C (375°F), Gas Mark 5, for 40 minutes until golden and bubbling. Serve with a green salad.

spinach & potato tortilla

Cost **££**
Timing
Serves **4**

what you need

- 3 tablespoons olive oil
- 2 onions, finely chopped
- 250 g (8 oz) cooked potatoes, peeled and cut into 1 cm (½ inch) cubes
- 2 garlic cloves, finely chopped
- 200 g (7 oz) cooked spinach, drained thoroughly and roughly chopped
- 4 tablespoons finely chopped (drained) roasted red peppers (in oil, from a jar)
- 5 eggs
- 3–4 tablespoons grated Manchego-style cheese
- salt and pepper

what you do

1. Heat the oil in a nonstick, ovenproof frying pan and add the onions and potatoes. Cook over a medium heat for 3–4 minutes or until the vegetables have softened but not coloured, turning and stirring often. Add the garlic, spinach and peppers and stir to mix well.

2. Beat the eggs lightly in a jug and season well with salt and pepper. Pour the eggs into the frying pan, shaking the pan so that the egg mixture is evenly spread. Cook gently for 8–10 minutes or until the tortilla is set at the bottom.

3. Sprinkle over the grated cheese. Place the frying pan under a preheated medium-hot grill and cook for 3–4 minutes or until the top is set and golden.

4. Remove from the heat, cut into 4 wedges and serve warm or at room temperature.

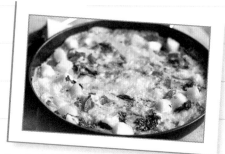

utternut squash & ricotta frittata

Cost
£

Timing

Serves
6

at you need

- tablespoon rapeseed oil
- red onion, thinly sliced
- 50 g (14½ oz) peeled and eseeded butternut squash, iced
- 3 eggs
- 1 tablespoon chopped thyme
- 2 tablespoons chopped sage
- 125 g (4 oz) ricotta cheese
- salt and pepper

what you do

1. Heat the oil in a large, deep, ovenproof frying pan over a medium-low heat, add the onion and butternut squash, then cover loosely and cook gently, stirring frequently, for 18–20 minutes or until softened and golden.

2. Lightly beat the eggs, thyme, sage and ricotta together in a jug, season well with salt and pepper and then pour evenly over the butternut squash. Cook for a further 2–3 minutes until the egg mixture is almost set, stirring occasionally with a heat-resistant rubber spatula to prevent the base from burning.

3. Slide the pan under a preheated medium-hot grill and grill for 3–4 minutes or until the top is set and the frittata is golden. Slice into 6 wedges and serve hot.

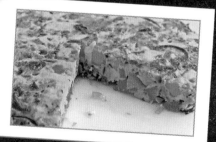

kedgeree-style rice with spinach

Cost
££

Timing

Serves
4

what you need

- 250 g (8 oz) smoked haddock fillets
- 125 g (4 oz) frozen peas
- 150 ml (¼ pint) boiling water
- 250 g (8 oz) spinach leaves
- 500 g (1 lb) express rice
- 25 g (1 oz) butter
- ½ teaspoon garam masala
- pepper
- 3 tablespoons chopped parsley, to garnish (optional)

what you do

1. Place the haddock and peas in a frying pan, cover with the boiling water and bring to the boil. Reduce the heat, cover and simmer for 3–4 minutes, adding the spinach for the final minute of cooking.
2. Meanwhile, microwave the express rice for 5 minutes or according to the packet instructions. Drain the fish, spinach and peas and flake the fish. Return to the pan and add the butter, garam masala and rice, season with pepper and toss well. Serve sprinkled with parsley, if liked.

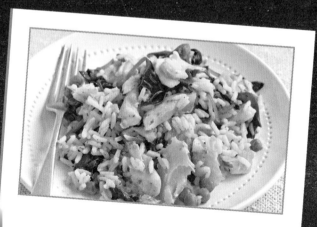

barley & ginger risotto with butternut squash

 Cost ££
 Timing ❶❶❶
 Serves 2

what you do

1. Cut the squash into 2 cm (¾ inch) cubes, discarding the skin and any seeds. Put in an ovenproof casserole with the onion and oil and stir to mix. Bake, covered, in a preheated oven 180°C (350°F), Gas Mark 4, for 30 minutes.
2. Stir in the garlic, pearl barley, rosemary, ginger and stock. Return to the oven, uncovered, and bake for a further 50 minutes. Stir the risotto occasionally during cooking until the barley is tender, adding a little more water if the consistency runs dry.
3. Remove the rosemary stalks. Season the risotto with plenty of pepper and stir in the soured cream. Spoon into bowls and serve sprinkled with cheese, if liked.

what you need

- 600 g (1 lb 2 oz) butternut squash
- 1 onion, chopped
- 1 tablespoon olive or sunflower oil
- 2 garlic cloves, thinly sliced
- 150 g (5 oz) pearl barley
- 2 large sprigs of rosemary
- 2 cm (¾ inch) piece of fresh root ginger, peeled and chopped
- 300 ml (½ pint) Vegetable Stock (see page 164)
- 4 tablespoons low-fat soured cream
- pepper
- grated Parmesan-style cheese, to serve (optional)

lemon & herb risotto

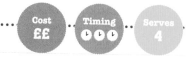

what you need

Cost ££   **Timing** ●●●   **Serves** 4

- 1 tablespoon olive oil
- 3 shallots, finely chopped
- 2 garlic cloves, finely chopped
- 1 head of celery, finely chopped
- 1 courgette, finely diced
- 1 carrot, finely diced
- 300 g (10 oz) arborio rice
- 1.2 litres (2 pints) hot Vegetable Stock (see page 164)
- good handful of fresh, mixed and roughly chopped herbs, such as tarragon, parsley, chives and dill
- 100 g (3½ oz) butter
- 1 tablespoon finely grated lemon rind
- 100 g (3½ oz) Parmesan-style cheese, grated
- salt and pepper

what you do

1. Heat the oil in a heavy-based saucepan and add the shallots, garlic, celery, courgette and carrot and fry gently for 4 minutes or until the vegetables have softened. Add the rice and turn up the heat. Stir-fry for 2–3 minutes.
2. Add a ladleful of hot Vegetable Stock followed by half of the mixed herbs and season well with salt and pepper. Reduce the heat to medium-low and add the remaining stock, 1 ladleful at a time, stirring constantly until each amount is absorbed and the rice is just firm to the bite but cooked through.
3. Remove from the heat and gently stir in the remaining herbs, the butter, lemon rind and cheese. Place the lid on the pan and allow to sit for 2–3 minutes, during which time it will become creamy and oozy. Serve immediately, sprinkled with pepper.

mixed bean & tomato chilli

Cost
£

Timing

Serves
1

what you do

1. Heat the oil in a heavy-based saucepan and add the onion and garlic. Stir-fry for 3–4 minutes, then add the chilli flakes, cumin and cinnamon.
2. Stir-fry for 2–3 minutes, then stir in the tomatoes. Bring to the boil, reduce the heat to medium and simmer gently for 10 minutes.
3. Stir in all the beans (and chilli sauce) and cook for 3–4 minutes until warmed through. Season well with salt and pepper and ladle into 4 bowls to serve.
4. Top each serving with a tablespoon of soured cream, garnish with chopped coriander and serve immediately with corn tortillas.

what you need

- 2 tablespoons olive oil
- 1 onion, finely chopped
- 4 garlic cloves, crushed
- 1 teaspoon dried chilli flakes
- 2 teaspoons ground cumin
- 1 teaspoon ground cinnamon
- 400 g (13 oz) can chopped tomatoes
- 400 g (13 oz) can mixed beans, rinsed and drained
- 400 g (13 oz) can red kidney beans in chilli sauce
- salt and pepper

To serve
- 4 tablespoons low-fat soured cream
- 25 g (1 oz) finely chopped fresh coriander, to garnish
- warmed corn tortillas

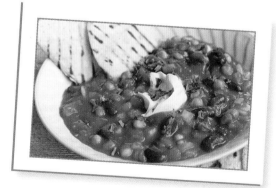

cauliflower & chickpea curry

Cost
£

Timing

Serves
4

what you need

- 1 tablespoon groundnut oil
- 8 spring onions, cut into 5 cm (2 inch) lengths
- 2 teaspoons grated garlic
- 2 teaspoons ground ginger
- 2 tablespoons medium curry powder
- 300 g (10 oz) cauliflower florets
- 1 red pepper, cored, deseeded and diced
- 1 yellow pepper, cored, deseeded and diced
- 400 g (13 oz) can chopped tomatoes
- 400 g (13 oz) can chickpeas, rinsed and drained
- salt and pepper

To serve
- Boiled Rice (optional) (see page 167)
- mint raita (optional)

what you do

1. Heat the oil in a large, nonstick frying pan over a medium heat. Add the spring onions and stir-fry for 2–3 minutes. Add the garlic, ginger and curry powder and stir-fry for 20–30 seconds until fragrant. Add the cauliflower and peppers and stir-fry for a further 2–3 minutes.
2. Stir in the tomatoes and bring to the boil. Cover, reduce the heat a little and simmer for 10 minutes, stirring occasionally. Add the chickpeas, season to taste with salt and pepper and bring back to the boil.
3. Remove from the heat and serve immediately with boiled rice and mint raita, if liked.

Variation
For broccoli and black-eyed bean curry, replace the cauliflower with 300 g (10 oz) broccoli florets and the chickpeas with a 400 g (13 oz) can black-eyed beans.

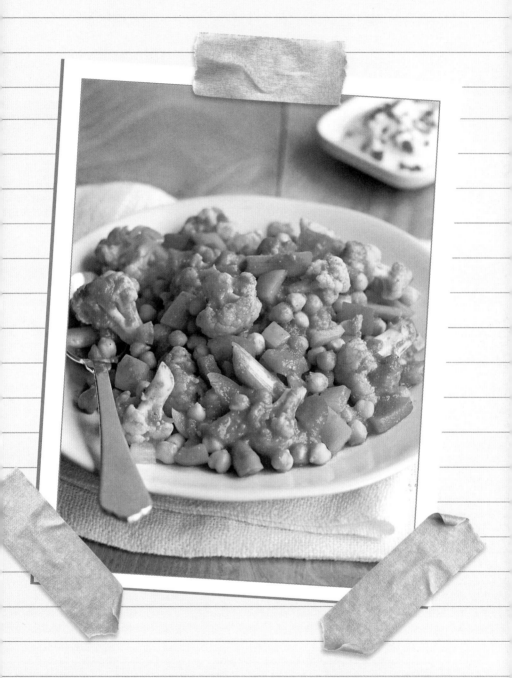

vegetable curry with rice

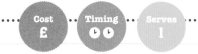
what you need

- 2 tablespoons vegetable oil
- 1 onion, roughly chopped
- 600 g (1 lb 3 oz) mixed chopped vegetables, such as carrots, leeks, swede, potato, cauliflower and broccoli
- 2 garlic cloves, chopped
- 2.5 cm (1 inch) piece of fresh root ginger, peeled and chopped
- 4 tablespoons medium-hot curry paste, such as rogan josh or balti
- 400 g (13 oz) can chopped tomatoes
- 400 ml (14 fl oz) Vegetable Stock (see page 164)
- Boiled Rice (see page 167), to serve

what you do

1. Heat the oil in a large frying pan and cook the onion and mixed vegetables over a medium heat for about 10 minutes, stirring frequently, until lightly coloured and beginning to soften. Stir in the garlic and ginger and cook for a further 2 minutes, then add the curry paste and stir over the heat for 1 minute to cook the spices.
2. Pour in the chopped tomatoes and stock, then bring to the boil, reduce the heat and simmer gently for about 15 minutes, stirring occasionally, until the curry has thickened slightly and the vegetables are tender. Serve spooned over boiled rice.

vegetable, fruit & nut biryani

Cost
£

Timing

Serves
4

what you need

- 250 g (8 oz) basmati rice
- ½ cauliflower, broken into florets
- 2 tablespoons vegetable oil
- 2 large sweet potatoes, peeled and cut into cubes
- 1 large onion, sliced
- 3 tablespoons hot curry paste
- ½ teaspoon ground turmeric
- 2 teaspoons mustard seeds
- 300 ml (½ pint) Vegetable Stock (see page 164)
- 250 g (8 oz) fine green beans, topped, tailed and cut in half
- 100 g (3½ oz) sultanas
- 6 tablespoons chopped fresh coriander
- 50 g (2 oz) cashew nuts, lightly toasted
- salt

To serve
- poppadums
- raita

what you do

1. Bring a large saucepan of lightly salted water to the boil and cook the rice for 5 minutes. Add the cauliflower and cook with the rice for a further 10 minutes or until both are tender, then drain.
2. Meanwhile, heat the oil in a large, heavy-based frying pan and cook the sweet potatoes and onion over a medium heat, stirring occasionally, for 10 minutes until browned and tender. Add the curry paste, turmeric and mustard seeds and cook, stirring, for a further 2 minutes.
3. Pour in the stock and add the green beans. Bring to the boil, then reduce the heat and simmer for 5 minutes. Stir in the drained rice and cauliflower, the sultanas, coriander and cashew nuts and simmer for a further 2 minutes. Spoon on to serving plates and serve with poppadums and raita.

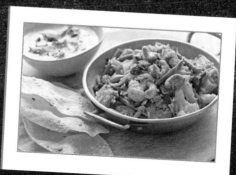

baked sweet potatoes

what you need

Cost £

Timing ▶ ▶ ▶

Serves 4

- 4 sweet potatoes, about 250 g (8 oz) each, scrubbed
- 200 ml (7 fl oz) low-fat soured cream
- 2 spring onions, finely chopped
- 1 tablespoon snipped chives
- 50 g (2 oz) butter
- salt and pepper

what you do

1. Put the potatoes on a baking tray and roast in a preheated oven, 220°C (425°F), Gas Mark 7, for 45–50 minutes until cooked through.
2. Combine the soured cream, spring onions, chives and salt and pepper in a bowl.
3. Cut the baked potatoes in half lengthways, top with the butter and spoon over the soured cream mixture. Serve immediately.

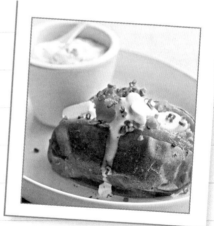

caribbean chicken with rice & peas

Cost ££

Timing

Serves 2

what you need

- 2 teaspoons jerk seasoning
- 1 teaspoon peeled and grated fresh root ginger
- juice of 1 lime
- 2 boneless, skinless chicken breasts, about 150 g (5 oz) each
- 3 tablespoons vegetable oil
- 1 small onion, chopped
- 1 garlic clove, crushed
- 150 g (5 oz) long-grain rice
- 175 ml (6 fl oz) Chicken Stock (see page 165)
- 175 ml (6 fl oz) coconut milk
- 200 g (7 oz) can red kidney beans, rinsed and drained
- 50 g (2 oz) frozen or canned sweetcorn
- few thyme sprigs, plus extra to garnish
- lime wedges, to serve

what you do

1. Mix together the jerk seasoning, ginger and lime juice in a non-metallic bowl. Cut a few slashes across each chicken breast and coat in the mixture. Heat 2 tablespoons of the oil in a frying pan, add the chicken and cook over a medium heat for 15-20 minutes, turning occasionally, until cooked through.

2. Meanwhile, heat the remaining oil in a saucepan, add the onion and garlic and cook for 2 minutes until slightly softened. Add the rice, stock and coconut milk and bring to the boil, then reduce the heat, cover and simmer for 15-20 minutes until the liquid has been absorbed and the rice is tender, adding the kidney beans, sweetcorn and thyme sprigs for the final 5 minutes.

3. Slice the chicken and serve with the rice mixture and lime wedges, garnished with a few sprigs of thyme.

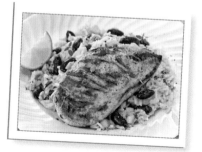

chicken & spinach stew

Cost
££

Timing

Serves
4

what you need

- 625 g (1¼ lb) boneless, skinless chicken thighs, thinly sliced
- 2 teaspoons ground cumin
- 1 teaspoon ground ginger
- 2 tablespoons olive oil
- 1 tablespoon tomato purée
- 2 x 400 g (13 oz) cans cherry tomatoes
- 50 g (2 oz) raisins
- 250 g (8 oz) ready-cooked Puy lentils
- 1 teaspoon finely grated lemon rind
- 150 g (5 oz) baby spinach
- salt and pepper
- handful of chopped parsley, to garnish
- steamed couscous or Boiled Rice (see page 167), to serve

what you do

1. Mix the chicken with the ground spices until well coated. Heat the oil in a large saucepan or flameproof casserole, then add the chicken and cook for 2-3 minutes until lightly browned.
2. Stir in the tomato purée, tomatoes, raisins, lentils and lemon rind. Season with salt and pepper and simmer gently, stirring occasionally, for about 12 minutes until thickened slightly and the chicken is cooked.
3. Add the spinach and stir until wilted. Ladle the stew into serving bowls, then scatter with the parsley and serve with steamed couscous or rice.

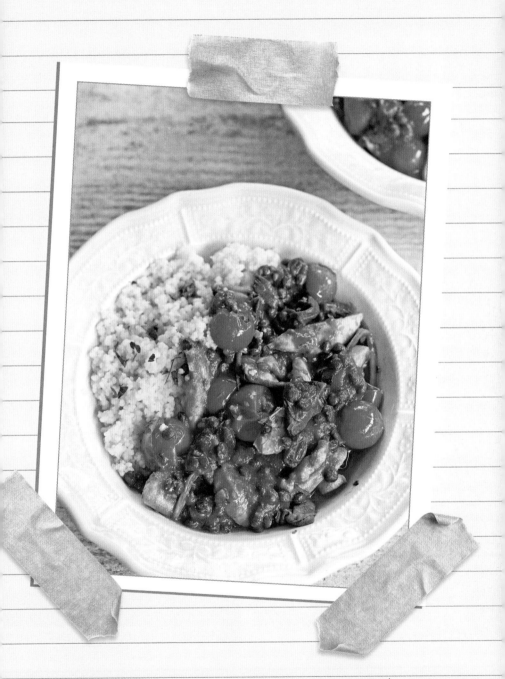

chicken jalfrezi

Cost
£

Timing

Serves
2

what you need

- 2 tablespoons sunflower oil
- 300 g (10 oz) boneless, skinless chicken breasts, cut into pieces
- 1 onion, cut into thin wedges
- 1 small green pepper, cored, deseeded and cut into chunks
- 1 green chilli, deseeded and finely chopped
- 1 teaspoon ground cumin
- 1 teaspoon garam masala
- 1½ teaspoons ground turmeric
- 2 tomatoes, cut into wedges
- 2 tablespoons natural yogurt
- 200 ml (7 fl oz) hot water
- warm naan bread, to serve

what you do

1. Heat the oil in a large frying pan, add the chicken, onion and green pepper and cook over a medium heat, stirring occasionally, for 10 minutes until chicken starts to turn golden. Add the chilli and spices and cook for 2–3 minutes, then stir in the tomatoes and cook for a further 3 minutes.
2. Stir in the yogurt, then pour in the hot water, cover and simmer very gently for 10 minutes until the chicken is cooked through and the flavours have infused, stirring occasionally and adding a little more water if necessary. Serve with warm naan bread to mop up the juices. Discard the cardamom pods. Serve the porridge in bowls topped with a dollop of natural yogurt, 100 g (3½ oz) chopped pitted dates and sliced banana.

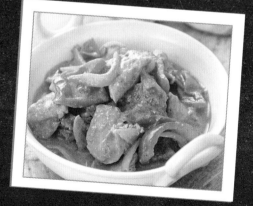

chicken shawarma

what you need

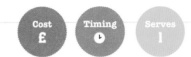

Cost £

Timing ◔

Serves 1

- 1 teaspoon olive or vegetable oil
- ½ onion, thinly sliced
- 200 g (7 oz) boneless, skinless chicken thighs, cut into large pieces
- 1 teaspoon shawarma spice
- 1 wholemeal pitta bread
- 1 tablespoon tahini

- 1 teaspoon clear honey
- 1 teaspoon white or red wine vinegar
- 4 teaspoons hot water
- 1 Little Gem lettuce
- 1 gherkin, sliced
- salt and pepper

what you do

1. Heat the oil in a small frying pan and fry the onion for 3 minutes until softened. Add the chicken and fry for a further 5 minutes, stirring frequently until the chicken is cooked through. Stir in the shawarma spice and cook for a further 1 minute.
2. Lightly toast the pitta bread. Mix the tahini with the honey, vinegar and hot water in a small bowl. Season lightly with salt and pepper.
3. Shred the lettuce on a serving plate and pile the chicken mixture on top. Scatter with the gherkin and spoon over the tahini dressing. Serve with the toasted pitta bread.

jambalaya with chorizo & peppers

Cost **££** Timing ⏱⏱ Serves **9**

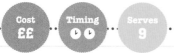

what you do

what you need

- 150 g (5 oz) brown basmati rice
- 1 tablespoon olive oil
- 1 onion, chopped
- 1 red pepper, cored, deseeded and chopped
- 1 yellow pepper, cored, deseeded and chopped
- 150 g (5 oz) spicy chorizo sausage, diced
- 400 g (13 oz) can chopped tomatoes
- ¼ teaspoon ground allspice
- 1 teaspoon caster sugar
- 100g (3½ oz) frozen peas
- salt and pepper

1. Cook the rice in a large saucepan of boiling water for about 25 minutes until tender. Drain the rice.
2. Meanwhile, heat the oil in a frying pan and gently fry the onion, peppers and chorizo for 10–15 minutes, stirring occasionally, until softened and beginning to brown.
3. Stir in the tomatoes, allspice and sugar and cook for 5 minutes until the tomato juices are reduced. Stir in the cooked rice and peas and season to taste with salt and pepper. Heat through for 5 minutes, then serve.

HEALTHY TIP
Stick to use-by dates.
Food poisoning is a daily danger for students preparing food in less than salubrious surroundings. Lower your chances by sticking to the advice on food labels – if its use by today don't let it fester in the fridge for another couple of nights.

chicken burgers with tomato salsa

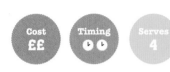

Cost **££**

Timing **◐ ◐**

Serves **4**

what you need

- 1 garlic clove, crushed
- 3 spring onions, thinly sliced
- 1 tablespoon Pesto (see page 168)
- 2 tablespoons chopped mixed herbs, such as parsley, tarragon and thyme
- 375 g (12 oz) minced chicken
- 2 sun-dried tomatoes, finely chopped
- 1 teaspoon olive oil

Tomato salsa
- 250 g (8 oz) cherry tomatoes, quartered
- 1 red chilli, deseeded and finely chopped
- 1 tablespoon chopped fresh coriander
- finely grated rind and juice of 1 lime

To serve
- 4 bread rolls
- salad leaves

1. Mix together all the burger ingredients, except the oil. Divide the mixture into 4 and form each portion into a burger. Cover and chill for 30 minutes.
2. Combine all the salsa ingredients in a bowl. Cover and set aside.
3. Brush the burgers with the oil and cook under a preheated high grill or on a preheated barbecue for about 3–4 minutes each side until cooked through. Serve each burger in a bread roll with the tomato salsa and some salad leaves.

Variation
For chilli and coriander chicken burgers with mango salsa, make the burgers as above, replacing the sun-dried tomatoes with a finely chopped deseeded red chilli (and using coriander pesto in place of the standard pesto). Serve with a salsa made from 1 peeled and stoned large ripe mango, 1 small red onion and 1 deseeded red chilli, all finely chopped, then mixed with 2 tablespoons chopped fresh coriander, 2 tablespoons chopped mint leaves, juice of 1 lime and 2 teaspoons olive oil.

chicken fajitas with no-chilli salsa

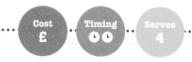

Cost **£**

Timing **◑ ◑**

Serves **4**

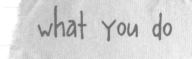

what you need

- ½ teaspoon ground coriander
- ½ teaspoon ground cumin
- ½ teaspoon paprika
- 1 garlic clove, crushed
- 3 tablespoons chopped fresh coriander
- 375 g (12 oz) boneless, skinless chicken breasts
- 1 tablespoon olive oil
- 4 soft flour tortillas

Salsa
- 3 ripe tomatoes, finely chopped
- 3 tablespoons chopped fresh coriander
- ⅛ cucumber, finely chopped
- 1 tablespoon olive oil

Guacamole
- 1 large ripe avocado, peeled, stoned and chopped
- finely grated rind and juice of ½ lime
- sweet chilli sauce, to taste (optional)

what you do

1. To make the chicken fajitas, place all the ground spices, garlic and chopped coriander in a mixing bowl. Cut the chicken into bite-sized strips and toss in the oil, then add to the spices and toss to coat lightly in the spice mixture.

2. Make the salsa. Mix the tomatoes, coriander and cucumber in a bowl and drizzle over the oil. Transfer to a serving bowl.

3. Make the guacamole. Mash the avocado in a bowl with the lime rind and juice and sweet chilli sauce, if using, until soft and rough-textured.

4. Heat a griddle pan or heavy-based frying pan until hot and cook the chicken for 3–4 minutes, turning occasionally, until golden and cooked through. Top the tortillas with the hot chicken strips, guacamole and salsa, and fold into quarters to serve.

pot roast chicken

This dish makes a delightful change from a traditional roast chicken. If you have any leftover chicken, mix with mayo and shredded lettuce for an easy sandwich filling.

Cost
£££

Timing
● ● ●

Serves
4

what you need

- 1.5 kg (3 lb) oven-ready chicken
- 25 g (1 oz) butter
- 2 tablespoons olive oil
- 1 onion, sliced
- 3 celery sticks, sliced
- 4–6 garlic cloves, crushed
- 250 ml (8 fl oz) dry white wine
- 3 bay leaves
- sprigs of thyme
- 150 g (5 oz) Puy lentils
- 2 tablespoons capers, drained
- 4 tablespoons chopped parsley
- 100 ml (3½ fl oz) half-fat crème fraîche
- salt and pepper

what you do

1. Season the chicken all over with salt and pepper. Melt the butter with the oil in a frying pan and fry the chicken on all sides. Transfer to a large, ovenproof casserole.
2. Fry the onion and celery in the pan juices for 6–8 minutes or until browned. Stir in the garlic, wine and herbs and pour over the chicken. Cover and bake in a preheated oven, 160°C (325°F), Gas Mark 3, for 1 hour.
3. Meanwhile, rinse the lentils and put them in a saucepan with plenty of water. Bring to the boil and boil for 10 minutes. Drain well.
4. Tip the lentils around the chicken and return to the oven for a further 45 minutes. Transfer the cooked chicken and lentil mixture to a warmed serving dish and cover. Remember to remove the bay leaves and thyme stalks before serving.
5. Mix the capers, parsley and crème fraîche together in a small pan and heat through gently, stirring. Serve with the carved chicken and the lentil mixture.

roasted lemony chicken with courgettes

Cost
£

Timing

Serves
2

what you need

- 4 chicken thighs, about 100 g (3½ oz) each
- finely grated rind of 1 lemon
- 1 garlic clove, crushed, plus 2 whole cloves, unpeeled
- 4 tablespoons olive oil
- 375 g (12 oz) new potatoes, halved if large
- 1 red onion, cut into wedges
- 1 courgette, thickly sliced
- 1 tablespoon thyme leaves, plus a few sprigs to garnish
- salt and pepper

what you do

1. Cut a few slashes across each chicken thigh. Mix together the lemon rind, crushed garlic and 2 tablespoons of the oil in a bowl, then rub this mixture over the chicken thighs, pushing it into the slashes.
2. Place the chicken in a roasting tin with the potatoes and season with salt and pepper. Roast in a preheated oven, 220°C (425°F), Gas Mark 7, for 10 minutes.
3. Add the onion, courgette, unpeeled garlic cloves and thyme leaves to the tin and drizzle with the remaining oil. Return to the oven and roast for a further 15 minutes or until the chicken is golden and cooked through and the vegetables are tender.
4. Squeeze the soft garlic over the chicken and vegetables, discarding the skin, and serve garnished with thyme sprigs.

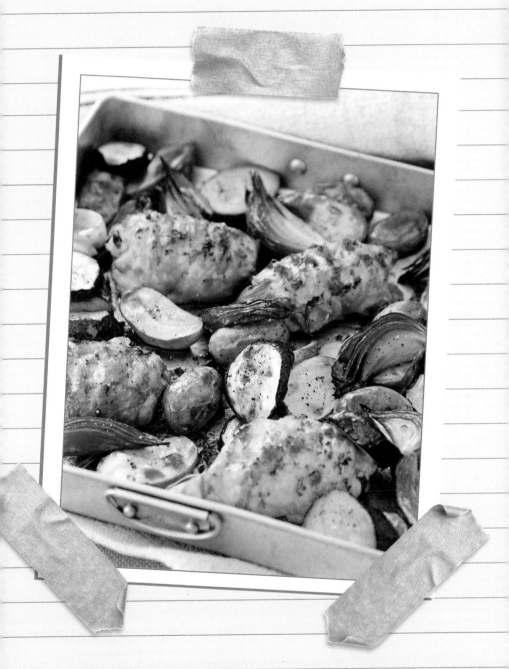

warm chicken, med veg & bulgar wheat salad

Cost
£

Timing

Serves
4

what you do

1. Heat 5 tablespoons of the oil in a large frying pan, add the courgette, onion, red pepper, aubergine and garlic and cook over a high heat for 15–20 minutes, stirring regularly until golden and softened.
2. Meanwhile, cook the bulgar wheat in a saucepan of lightly salted boiling water for 15 minutes until tender.
3. While the bulgar wheat is cooking, brush the remaining oil over the chicken breasts and season well with salt and pepper. Heat a large griddle pan until smoking, then add the chicken and cook over a high heat for 4–5 minutes on each side or until golden and cooked through. Remove from the heat and thinly slice diagonally.
4. Drain the bulgar wheat. Place in a large bowl, toss with the parsley and season with salt and pepper. Add the hot vegetables and chicken, toss together and serve.

what you need

- 6 tablespoons olive oil
- 1 large courgette, cut into thick slices
- 1 large red onion, cut into thin wedges
- 1 red pepper, cored, deseeded and cut into chunks
- ½ small aubergine, cut into small chunks
- 1 garlic clove, thinly sliced
- 150 g (5 oz) bulgar wheat
- 4 chicken breasts, about 150 g (5 oz) each
- 4 tablespoons chopped parsley
- salt and pepper

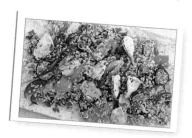

oven-baked turkey & gruyère burgers

what you need

Cost
£££

Timing

Serves
4

- 1 small red onion
- 500g (1lb) minced turkey
- ½ teaspoon dried thyme or oregano
- 90 g (3¼ oz) Gruyère cheese
- 1 teaspoon olive or sunflower oil

- 2 seeded buns
- 25 g (1 oz) walnuts, finely chopped
- 4 tablespoons mayonnaise
- 50 g (2 oz) watercress
- salt and pepper

what you do

1. Thinly slice half of the onion and reserve. Finely chop the remainder and mix in a bowl with the minced turkey, dried herbs and a little salt and pepper. Divide into 4 even-sized portions. Cut the Gruyère into 4 pieces and push a piece into the centre of each portion of minced turkey. Flatten out into burger shapes.
2. Brush a baking sheet with a little of the oil and place the burgers on top. Brush the burgers with the remaining oil, then bake in a preheated oven, 200°C (400°F), Gas Mark 6, for 20 minutes, turning the burgers halfway through cooking.
3. Halve the seeded buns. Stir the walnuts into the mayonnaise and season with pepper. Place the burgers on the bun bases and top with the walnut mayonnaise, watercress and sliced onion. Top with the burger lids and serve.

swedish meatballs

what you do

1. Make the cranberry glaze. Combine the cranberry sauce, stock, chilli sauce and lemon juice in a small saucepan and heat slowly until smooth, stirring, then simmer gently for 5 minutes. Remove from the heat and set aside.

2. Meanwhile, put the minced veal and pork in a food processor with the onion, garlic, breadcrumbs, egg yolk, parsley and a little salt and pepper, and process until the mixture forms a fairly smooth paste that clings together.

3. Scoop teaspoonfuls of the paste and roll them into small balls between the palms of your hands.

4. Heat the oil in a large, heavy-based frying pan and fry half of the meatballs, turning occasionally, for 8-10 minutes until golden. Drain and fry the remainder. Return all the meatballs to the pan and add the cranberry glaze. Cook gently for 2-3 minutes until hot. Serve immediately.

what you need

- 300 g (10 oz) lean minced veal (or minced beef if preferred)
- 200 g (7 oz) lean minced pork
- 1 small onion, chopped
- 1 garlic clove, crushed
- 25 g (1 oz) breadcrumbs
- 1 egg yolk
- 3 tablespoons chopped flat leaf parsley
- 2 tablespoons vegetable oil
- salt and pepper

Cranberry glaze
- 150 g (5 oz) good-quality cranberry sauce
- 100 ml (3½ fl oz) Chicken or Vegetable Stock (see page 165 or 164)
- 2 tablespoons sweet chilli sauce
- 1 tablespoon lemon juice

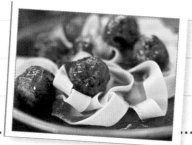

steak meatloaf

what you do

1. Scatter the red peppers and onion in a roasting tin and drizzle with the oil. Cook in a preheated oven, 200°C (400°F), Gas Mark 6, for 30 minutes until lightly roasted, then remove and chop. Reduce the oven temperature to 160°C (325°F), Gas Mark 3.
2. Use some bacon rashers to line the base and long sides of a 1 kg (2 lb) loaf tin, overlapping them slightly and letting the ends overhang the sides. Finely chop the rest of the bacon.
3. Mix together both minced meats, the chopped bacon, roasted vegetables, herbs, Worcestershire sauce, tomato paste, breadcrumbs, egg and salt and pepper.
4. Pack the mixture evenly into the tin and fold the ends of the bacon over the filling. Cover with foil, place in a roasting tin and pour in 2 cm (¾ inch) boiling water. Cook in the oven for 2 hours or until cooked through.
5. To serve hot, remove from the oven and leave the meatloaf in the tin for 15 minutes, then invert on to a serving plate. To serve cold, cool it in the tin, then remove, wrap in foil and refrigerate before serving.

what you need

- 2 red peppers, cored, deseeded and cut into chunks
- 1 red onion, sliced
- 3 tablespoons olive oil
- 300 g (10 oz) thin-cut streaky bacon rashers
- 500 g (1 lb) lean minced steak
- 250 g (8 oz) minced pork
- 2 tablespoons chopped oregano
- 2 tablespoons chopped flat leaf parsley
- 3 tablespoons Worcestershire sauce
- 2 tablespoons sun-dried tomato paste
- 50 g (2 oz) breadcrumbs
- 1 egg
- salt and pepper

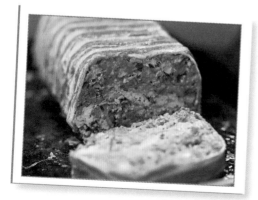

roast pork loin with creamy cabbage & leeks

Cost
£

Timing

Serves
2

what you need

- 1 teaspoon ground cumin
- 1 teaspoon ground coriander
- 500 g (1 lb) pork loin, trimmed of fat
- 3 tablespoons olive oil
- 300 g (10 oz) sweet potatoes, peeled and chopped
- 250 g (8 oz) Savoy cabbage, shredded
- 3 leeks, trimmed, cleaned and sliced
- 3 tablespoons low-fat soured cream
- 2 teaspoons wholegrain mustard

what you do

1. Mix together the spices in a bowl, then rub over the pork. Heat 1 tablespoon of the oil in an ovenproof frying pan, add the pork and cook until browned on all sides. Transfer to a preheated oven, 180°C (350°F), Gas Mark 4, and cook for 20–25 minutes or until cooked through. Leave to rest for 2 minutes.
2. Meanwhile, cook the sweet potatoes in a saucepan of boiling water for 12–15 minutes until tender, adding the cabbage and leeks 3–4 minutes before the end of the cooking time. Drain well.
3. Heat the remaining oil in a frying pan, add the drained vegetables and fry for 7–8 minutes, stirring occasionally, until starting to turn golden. Stir in the soured cream and mustard.
4. Slice the pork and serve on top of the vegetables.

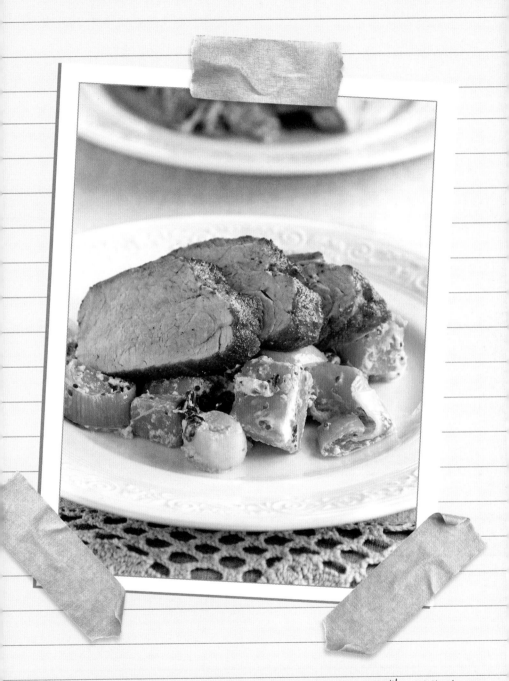

garlicky pork with warm butter bean salad

what you need

Cost ££ **Timing** 🕐 **Serves** 4

- 4 tablespoons olive oil
- 2 garlic cloves, crushed
- 4 lean pork chops or steaks, about 150 g (5 oz) each
- salt and pepper

Salad
- 2 tablespoons olive oil
- 2 x 400 g (13 oz) cans butter beans, rinsed and drained
- 12 cherry tomatoes, halved
- 150 ml (¼ pint) Chicken Stock (see page 169)
- juice of 2 lemons
- 2 handfuls of parsley, chopped

what you do

1. Mix together the oil and garlic in a bowl, then season with salt and pepper. Place the pork on a foil-lined grill rack and spoon over the garlicky oil. Cook under a preheated medium grill for about 10 minutes, turning occasionally, until golden and cooked through.
2. Meanwhile, make the salad. Heat the oil in a large frying pan, add the butter beans and tomatoes and heat through for a few minutes. Add the stock, lemon juice and parsley and season with salt and pepper. Serve with the grilled chops or steaks.

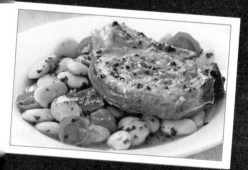

one-pan spiced pork

Cost	Timing	Serves
£		4

what You do

1. Snip through the fat on the rind of the pork chops so that they do not curl up during cooking. Place them in a large roasting tin with the parsnips, squash and apples.

2. Crush the fennel and coriander seeds using a pestle and mortar, then mix with the garlic, turmeric, oil and honey. Season with salt and pepper, then brush the mixture over the pork and vegetables.

3. Cook in a preheated oven, 190°C (375°F), Gas Mark 5, for 35–40 minutes, turning the vegetables once, until golden brown and tender. Spoon on to plates and serve immediately.

what You need

- 4 loin pork chops, about 175 g (6 oz) each
- 3 parsnips, cut into chunks
- 1 butternut squash, peeled, deseeded and thickly sliced
- 2 red-skinned dessert apples, cored and quartered
- 1 teaspoon fennel seeds
- 2 teaspoons coriander seeds
- 2 garlic cloves, chopped
- 1 teaspoon ground turmeric
- 3 tablespoons olive oil
- 1 tablespoon clear honey
- salt and pepper

HEALTHY TIP

Keep tabs on your alcohol units.

A cheeky pint after lectures and a few midweek drinks — it adds up. There are plenty of apps around that will tally up your drinks to help you keep on top of your recommended alcohol intake.

spicy sausage bake

what you need

Cost
££

Timing
◗ ◗ ◗

Serves
2

- 450 g (14½ oz) Italian sausages
- 2 tablespoons olive oil
- 1 large red onion, sliced
- 2 x 400 g (13 oz) cans chopped tomatoes
- 2 tablespoons chopped oregano
- 400 g (13 oz) can red kidney beans, rinsed and drained
- 200 g (7 oz) dried fusilli pasta
- 175 g (6 oz) fontina cheese, grated
- salt

what you do

1. Slice each sausage into quarters. Heat the oil in a large, heavy-based frying pan and gently fry the sausages and onion for about 10 minutes until golden, gently shaking the pan frequently.
2. Add the tomatoes, oregano and red kidney beans. Reduce the heat to its lowest setting, cover and cook gently for 10 minutes.
3. Meanwhile, cook the pasta in a large saucepan of lightly salted boiling water for about 10 minutes or until just tender. Drain and tip into the frying pan. Add half of the cheese and toss the ingredients together until mixed.
4. Tip the mixture into a 1.5 litre (2½ pint) shallow, ovenproof dish and scatter with the remaining cheese. Bake in a preheated oven, 200°C (400°F), Gas Mark 6, for 20–25 minutes or until the cheese is melting and golden.

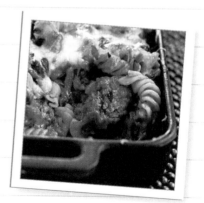

cheesy pork with parsnip purée

Cost ££ **Timing** ● ● **Serves** 4

what you need

- 4 lean pork steaks, about 125 g (4 oz) each
- 1 teaspoon olive oil
- 50 g (2 oz) crumbly cheese, such as Wensleydale or Cheshire, crumbled
- 1½ teaspoons chopped sage
- 75 g (3 oz) fresh granary breadcrumbs
- 1 egg yolk, beaten
- pepper
- steamed green beans or cabbage, to serve

Parsnip purée
- 625 g (1¼ lb) parsnips, chopped
- 2 garlic cloves, peeled
- 3 tablespoons half-fat crème fraîche

1. Season the pork steaks with plenty of pepper. Heat the oil in a nonstick frying pan, add the pork steaks and fry for 2 minutes on each side until browned, then transfer to an ovenproof dish.

2. Mix together the cheese, sage, breadcrumbs and egg yolk. Divide the mixture into 4 and use to top each of the pork steaks, pressing down gently. Cook in a preheated oven, 200 °C (400 °F), Gas Mark 6, for 12-15 minutes until the topping is golden.

3. Meanwhile, make the parsnip purée. Place the parsnips and garlic in a saucepan of boiling water and cook for 10-12 minutes until tender. Drain, then mash with the crème fraîche and plenty of pepper. Serve with the pork steaks and steamed green beans or cabbage.

Variation
For chicken with breaded tomato topping, replace the pork with 4 boneless, skinless chicken breasts. Brown and lay in an ovenproof dish, as above. Make the topping as above, replacing the sage with 4 chopped sun-dried tomatoes and ¼ teaspoon dried oregano. Bake as above and serve with the parsnip purée.

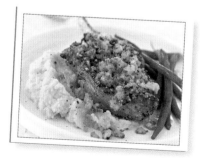

chorizo & ham eggs

Cost £

Timing ●

Serves 2

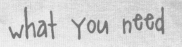

what you need

- 1 tablespoon olive oil
- 1 small red pepper, cored, deseeded and sliced
- 125 g (4 oz) chorizo sausage, thinly sliced
- 2 tomatoes, roughly chopped
- 50 g (2 oz) wafer-thin ham slices
- 2 handfuls of baby spinach leaves
- 2 large eggs
- warm crusty bread, to serve

what you do

1. Heat the oil in a frying pan, add the red pepper and chorizo and cook over a high heat for 2 minutes until golden. Add the tomatoes and cook for a further 2 minutes, then add the ham and spinach and cook, stirring occasionally, for 2 minutes.

2. Divide the mixture between 2 small, individual pans, if you have them (if not, continue to cook in one pan). Make wells in the tomato mixture and break an egg into each well. Cover and cook for 2–3 minutes over a medium heat until set. Serve with warm crusty bread to mop up the juices.

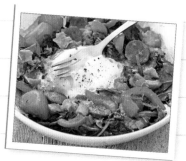

butter bean & chorizo stew

what you need

- 1 tablespoon olive oil
- 1 large onion, chopped
- 2 garlic cloves, crushed
- 200 g (7 oz) chorizo sausage, sliced
- 1 green pepper, cored, deseeded and chopped
- 1 red pepper, cored, deseeded and chopped
- 1 small glass of red wine
- 2 x 400 g (13 oz) cans butter beans, rinsed and drained
- 400 g (13 oz) can cherry tomatoes
- 1 tablespoon tomato purée
- salt and pepper
- chopped parsley, to garnish
- crusty bread, to serve (optional)

what you do

1. Heat the oil in a flameproof casserole, add the onion and garlic and fry for 1–2 minutes. Stir in the chorizo and fry until beginning to brown. Add the peppers and fry for 3 minutes.
2. Pour in the wine and allow it to bubble, then stir in the butter beans, tomatoes and tomato purée and season well with salt and pepper. Cover and simmer for 15 minutes, stirring occasionally.
3. Ladle into shallow bowls, sprinkle with the parsley to garnish and serve with crusty bread, if liked.

Variation

For garlic prawns with butter beans, cook the onion and garlic as above, then stir in 300 g (10 oz) raw peeled and deveined tiger prawns instead of the chorizo and fry until they just turn pink. Add the butter beans, 3 tablespoons half-fat crème fraîche and 2 handfuls of rocket and season well with salt and pepper. Heat through and serve.

west indian beef & bean stew

what You need

Cost
££

Timing

Serves
4–6

- 3 tablespoons sunflower oil
- 800 g (1 lb 12 oz) lean minced beef
- 6 whole cloves
- 1 onion, finely chopped
- 2 tablespoons medium curry powder
- 2 carrots, cut into 1 cm (½ inch) cubes
- 2 celery sticks, diced
- 1 tablespoon thyme leaves
- 2 garlic cloves, crushed
- 4 tablespoons tomato purée
- 600 ml (1 pint) beef stock
- 1 large potato, peeled and cut into 1 cm (½ inch) cubes
- 200 g (7 oz) can black beans, rinsed and drained
- 200 g (7 oz) can black-eyed beans, rinsed and drained
- salt and pepper
- lemon wedges, to serve

what You do

1. Heat the oil in a large, heavy-based saucepan, add the minced beef and fry, stirring, over a medium-high heat for 5–6 minutes or until browned. Add the cloves, onion and curry powder and cook for 2–3 minutes until the onion is beginning to soften, then stir in the carrots, celery, thyme, garlic and tomato purée.
2. Pour in the stock and stir well, then add the potato and beans and bring to the boil. Reduce the heat slightly and simmer for 20 minutes, uncovered, stirring occasionally, until the potatoes and beef are tender. Season to taste with salt and pepper. Ladle into bowls and serve with lemon wedges.

beef, pumpkin & prune stew

Cost
££

Timing

Serves
4

what you do

what you need

- 2 tablespoons olive oil
- 1 garlic clove, chopped
- 1 large onion, chopped
- 500 g (1 lb) peeled, deseeded and diced pumpkin
- 600 g (1 lb 3 oz) steak, such as sirloin, rump or frying, diced
- 2 teaspoons ground coriander
- 2 teaspoons ground cumin
- 150 g (5 oz) ready-to-eat pitted dried prunes
- 2 x 400 g (13 oz) cans chopped tomatoes
- 450 ml (¾ pint) beef stock
- 100 g (3½ oz) fresh coriander leaves, chopped

To serve
- steamed couscous (optional)
- natural yogurt

1. Heat the oil in a large saucepan or flameproof casserole, add the garlic, onion, pumpkin and steak and cook over a high heat for 5–10 minutes, stirring occasionally, until the beef is browned and the pumpkin is golden. Add the spices and cook for a further 1 minute.
2. Add the prunes, tomatoes and stock and bring to the boil, then reduce the heat, cover and simmer for 15 minutes, stirring occasionally, until the stew is thickened and the meat and vegetables are cooked through.
3. Serve with steamed couscous, if liked, scattered with chopped coriander and topped with spoonfuls of yogurt.

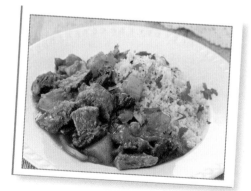

baked cod with tomatoes & olives

Cost
££

Timing
🕐

Serves
4

what you need

- 250 g (8 oz) cherry tomatoes, halved
- 100 g (3½ oz) pitted black olives
- 2 tablespoons capers, drained
- 4 thyme sprigs, plus extra to garnish
- 4 cod fillets, about 175 g (6 oz) each
- 2 tablespoons extra virgin olive oil
- 2 tablespoons balsamic vinegar
- salt and pepper
- mixed green leaf salad, to serve (optional)

what you do

1. Combine the tomatoes, olives, capers and thyme sprigs in a roasting tin. Nestle the cod fillets in the tin, drizzle over the oil and balsamic vinegar and season to taste with salt and pepper. Bake in a preheated oven, 200°C (400°F), Gas Mark 6, for 15 minutes until the fish is cooked through.
2. Transfer the fish, tomatoes and olives to plates. Spoon the pan juices over the fish. Garnish with thyme sprigs and serve immediately with a mixed green leaf salad, if liked.

Variation

For steamed cod with lemon, arrange a cod fillet on each of 4 x 30 cm (12 inch) squares of foil. Top each with ½ teaspoon finely grated lemon rind, a squeeze of lemon juice, 1 tablespoon extra virgin olive oil and salt and pepper to taste. Fold the edges of the foil together to form parcels, transfer to a baking sheet and cook in a preheated oven, 200°C (400°F), Gas Mark 6, for 15 minutes. Remove and leave to rest for 5 minutes. Open the parcels and serve sprinkled with chopped parsley.

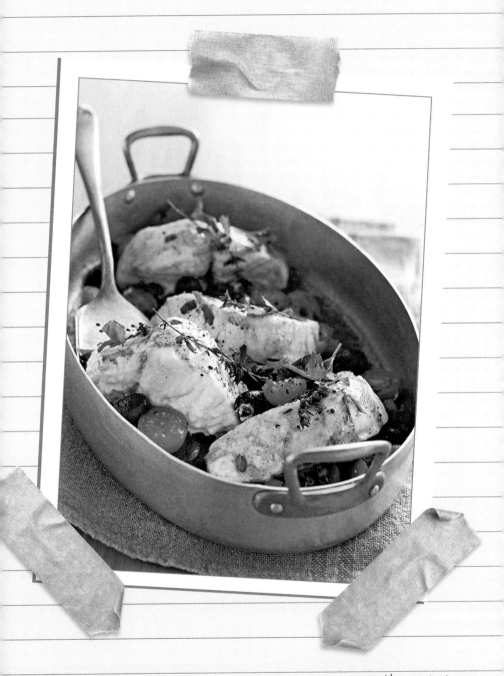

haddock with poached eggs

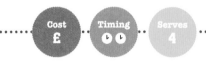
- 750 g (1½ lb) new potatoes
- 4 spring onions, sliced
- 2 tablespoons half-fat crème fraîche
- 75 g (3 oz) watercress
- 4 smoked haddock fillets, about 150 g (5 oz) each

- 150 ml (¼ pint) milk
- 1 bay leaf
- 4 eggs
- pepper

what you do

1. Place the potatoes in a saucepan of boiling water and cook for 12–15 minutes until tender. Drain, lightly crush with a fork, then stir through the spring onions, crème fraîche and watercress and season well with pepper. Keep warm.
2. Put the fish and milk in a large frying pan with the bay leaf. Bring to the boil, then cover and simmer for 5–6 minutes until the fish is cooked through. Remove from the heat and let stand while you poach the eggs.
3. Bring a saucepan of water to the boil, swirl the water with a spoon and crack in an egg, allowing the white to wrap around the yolk. Simmer for 3 minutes, then remove and keep warm. Repeat with the remaining eggs.
4. Serve the drained poached haddock on top of the crushed potatoes, topped with the poached eggs.

smoked mackerel kedgeree

Cost
£

Timing
⏱

Serves
4

what you need

- 3 large eggs
- 25 g (1 oz) butter
- 375 g (12 oz) smoked mackerel, skinned and flaked
- 375 g (12 oz) cooked basmati rice
- 1 teaspoon mild curry powder
- 4 tablespoons lemon juice
- 4 tablespoons chopped parsley

1. Place the eggs in a small saucepan of boiling water and cook them for 7 minutes. Drain, run under cold water, then shell them and cut into quarters.
2. Meanwhile, melt the butter in a frying pan, add the smoked mackerel, rice and curry powder and toss together until everything is warmed through and the rice is evenly coated.
3. Stir in the lemon juice, parsley and the quartered boiled eggs and serve immediately.

STUDENT TIP
Bag a bargain.
If you have space in your freezer, make the most of supermarket bargains and tuck them away for when the budget is straining.

quick tuna fishcakes

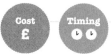

what you need

Cost	Timing	Serves
£	◑ ◑	4

- 250 g (8 oz) baking potatoes, peeled and diced
- 2 x 200 g (7 oz) cans tuna in olive oil, drained
- 50 g (2 oz) Cheddar cheese, grated
- 4 spring onions, finely chopped
- 1 small garlic clove, crushed
- 2 teaspoons dried thyme

- 1 small egg, beaten
- ½ teaspoon cayenne pepper
- 4 tablespoons plain flour
- vegetable oil, for frying
- salt and pepper

To serve
- mixed green salad
- mayonnaise

what you do

1. Cook the potatoes in a saucepan of lightly salted boiling water for 10 minutes or until tender. Drain well, mash and cool slightly.
2. Flake the tuna. Beat the tuna, cheese, spring onions, garlic, thyme and egg into the mashed potatoes. Season to taste with cayenne, salt and pepper.
3. Divide the mixture into 4 even portions and shape each one into a thick patty. Season the flour with salt and pepper, then dust the patties all over with the flour.
4. Heat a shallow layer of vegetable oil in a frying pan until hot, then fry the fishcakes for 5 minutes on each side or until crisp and golden. Serve hot with a mixed green salad and mayonnaise.

red salmon & roasted vegetables

what you need

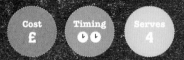

Cost
£

Timing
🕐🕐

Serves
4

- 1 aubergine, cut into bite-sized pieces
- 2 red peppers, cored, deseeded and cut into bite-sized pieces
- 2 red onions, quartered
- 1 garlic clove, crushed
- 4 tablespoons olive oil
- pinch of dried oregano
- 200 g (7 oz) can red salmon, drained and flaked
- 100 g (3½ oz) pitted black olives
- salt and pepper
- basil leaves, to garnish

what you do

1. Mix together the aubergine, red peppers, onions and garlic in a bowl with the oil and oregano and season well with salt and pepper. Spread the vegetables out in a single layer in a nonstick roasting tin and roast in a preheated oven, 220°C (425°F), Gas Mark 7, for 25 minutes or until the vegetables are just cooked.

2. Transfer the vegetables to a warmed serving dish and gently toss in the salmon and olives. Serve warm or at room temperature, garnished with basil leaves.

Accompaniment Tip

For rocket and cucumber couscous to serve with the salmon and vegetables, put 200 g (7 oz) instant couscous in a large, heatproof bowl. Season well with salt and pepper and pour over boiling hot water to just cover the couscous. Cover and leave to stand for 10–12 minutes until all the water has been absorbed. Meanwhile, finely chop 4 spring onions, halve, deseed and chop ½ cucumber and chop 75 g (3 oz) rocket. Fluff up the couscous grains with a fork and tip into a serving dish. Stir in the prepared ingredients along with 2 tablespoons olive oil and 1 tablespoon lemon juice. Toss well to mix, then serve with the salmon and vegetables.

Super Salads, Snacks and Sides

fattoush salad

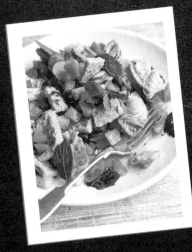

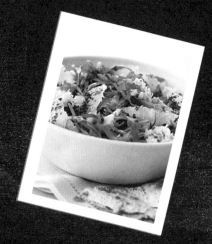

crab & grapefruit salad

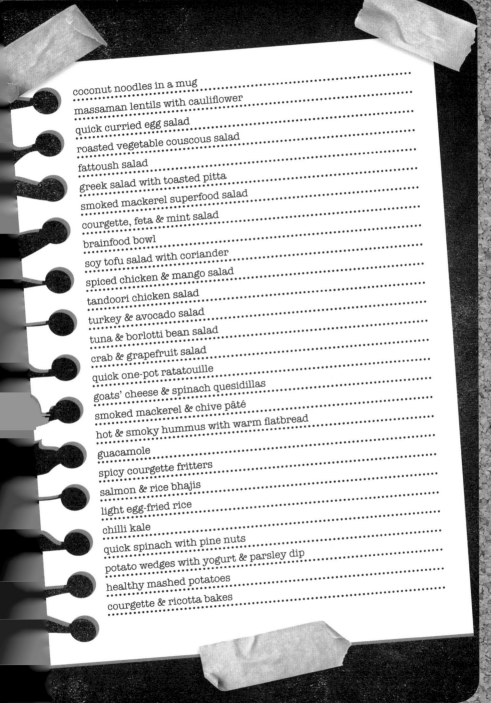

coconut noodles in a mug

massaman lentils with cauliflower

quick curried egg salad

roasted vegetable couscous salad

fattoush salad

greek salad with toasted pitta

smoked mackerel superfood salad

courgette, feta & mint salad

brainfood bowl

soy tofu salad with coriander

spiced chicken & mango salad

tandoori chicken salad

turkey & avocado salad

tuna & borlotti bean salad

crab & grapefruit salad

quick one-pot ratatouille

goats' cheese & spinach quesidillas

smoked mackerel & chive pâté

hot & smoky hummus with warm flatbread

guacamole

spicy courgette fritters

salmon & rice bhajis

light egg-fried rice

chilli kale

quick spinach with pine nuts

potato wedges with yogurt & parsley dip

healthy mashed potatoes

courgette & ricotta bakes

coconut noodles in a mug

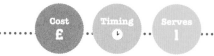

Cost
£

Timing
⏱

Serves
1

- 3 spring onions, thinly sliced
- 100 g (3½ oz) courgette, grated
- 1 teaspoon wok oil
- 100 ml (3½ fl oz) coconut milk
- ¼ teaspoon vegetable bouillon powder
- ½ teaspoon Thai spice powder, such as Thai 7 spice or Thai 5 spice

- good pinch of ground turmeric (optional)
- 75 ml (3 fl oz) boiling water
- 25 g (1 oz) vermicelli rice noodles
- 10 cashew nuts, roughly chopped

what you do

1. Mix together the spring onions, courgette and oil in a large, microwave-proof mug and microwave on medium power for 2 minutes.
2. Stir in the coconut milk, bouillon powder, Thai spice, turmeric, if using, and the boiling water. Microwave on medium power for 1 minute.
3. Break the noodles into the mug and stir to mix. Microwave on medium power for 1 minute. Stir again and microwave on medium power for a further 1½ minutes until the noodles are tender. Sprinkle with the cashew nuts and serve.

massaman lentils with cauliflower

Cost
£

Timing
🕐 🕐

Serves
2

what you need

- 150 g (5 oz) green lentils, rinsed and drained
- 20 g (¾ oz) butter
- 1 teaspoon olive oil
- 2 onions, sliced
- 1 large carrot, thinly sliced
- 1 small cauliflower or ½ large cauliflower, about 400 g (13 oz), cut into large florets
- 1 tablespoon Massaman curry paste
- 1 teaspoon light muscovado or caster sugar
- 1.5 cm (¾ inch) piece of fresh root ginger, peeled and grated
- 500 ml (17 fl oz) Vegetable Stock (see page 164)
- small handful of Thai basil, torn into pieces
- salt and pepper
- Boiled Rice (see page 167), to serve

what you do

1. Cook the lentils in a saucepan of boiling water for 15 minutes until softened but not falling apart. Drain well.
2. Meanwhile, melt the butter with the oil in a separate saucepan. Add the onions and carrot and fry gently for 5 minutes, stirring frequently. Add the cauliflower and fry for a further 5 minutes.
3. Stir in the curry paste, sugar, ginger and stock and bring to a gentle simmer. Cook very gently, stirring frequently, for 10 minutes until the cauliflower is tender.
4. Stir in the lentils and basil, season to taste with salt and pepper and then serve with boiled jasmine or long-grain rice.

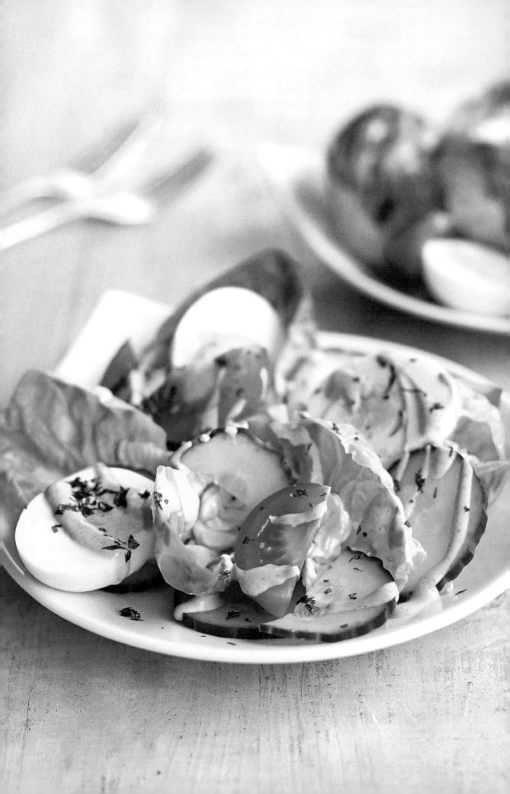

quick curried egg salad

what you need

- 8 hard-boiled eggs
- 4 tomatoes, cut into wedges
- 2 Little Gem lettuces, leaves separated
- ½ cucumber, sliced
- 200 ml (7 fl oz) natural yogurt
- 1 tablespoon mild curry powder
- 3 tablespoons tomato purée
- juice of 2 limes
- 6 tablespoons mayonnaise
- salt and pepper
- thyme leaves, to garnish

what you do

1. Shell, then halve the eggs and place on a large platter with the tomatoes, lettuce leaves and cucumber.
2. Mix the yogurt with the curry powder, tomato purée, lime juice and mayonnaise in a small bowl. Season the dressing with salt and pepper to taste, then pour it over the salad. Serve immediately, garnished with thyme leaves.

HEALTHY TIP

Snack attack.

Keep a cereal bar, piece of fresh fruit, some dried fruit or a snack bag of unsalted nuts or seeds in your bag for when you have a sudden energy slump. If there's a healthy snack on tap, you'll be less likely to raid the canteen for a doughnut.

roasted vegetable couscous salad

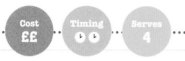

Cost	Timing	Serves
££	▶ ▶	4

what you do

1. Place all the vegetables on a large nonstick baking tray in a single layer. Drizzle with a little oil and season well with salt and pepper. Roast in a preheated oven, 200°C (400°F), Gas Mark 6, for 15–20 minutes or until the edges of the vegetables are just starting to char.
2. Meanwhile, put the couscous in a wide bowl and pour over enough boiling water to just cover. Season well. Cover with clingfilm and leave to stand, undisturbed, for 10 minutes or until all the liquid has been absorbed. Fluff up the grains with a fork and place on a wide, shallow serving platter.
3. Make the dressing by mixing together the orange juice, oil, cumin and cinnamon and season well with salt and pepper.
4. Fold the roasted vegetables, preserved lemons and herbs into the couscous, pour over the dressing and toss to mix well.
5. Scatter over the pine nuts, feta and pomegranate seeds and serve immediately.

what you need

- 1 red pepper, deseeded and cut into 2.5 cm (1 inch) pieces
- 1 yellow pepper, deseeded and cut into 2.5 cm (1 inch) pieces
- 1 medium aubergine, cut into 2.5 cm (1 inch) pieces
- 1 courgette, cut into 2.5 cm (1 inch) cubes
- 2 small red onions, cut into thick wedges
- olive oil, to drizzle
- 200 g (7 oz) couscous
- 6–8 preserved lemons, halved
- large handful of mint and coriander leaves, chopped
- 50 g (2 oz) pine nuts, toasted
- 150 g (5 oz) feta cheese, crumbled
- 100 g (3½ oz) pomegranate seeds
- salt and pepper

Dressing
- juice of 1 orange
- 5 tablespoons olive oil
- 1 teaspoon ground cumin
- 1 teaspoon ground cinnamon

fattoush salad

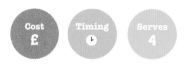

Cost	Timing	Serves
£	🕐	4

what you need

- 1 pitta bread, torn into small pieces
- 6 plum tomatoes, deseeded and roughly chopped
- 1 cucumber, peeled and roughly chopped
- 10 radishes, sliced
- 1 red onion, roughly chopped
- 1 small Little Gem lettuce, leaves separated
- small handful of fresh mint leaves

Dressing
- 200 ml (7 fl oz) olive oil
- juice of 3 lemons
- 1 garlic clove, crushed
- 2 teaspoons sumac or 2 teaspoons ground cumin
- salt and pepper

what you do

1. First make the dressing. Whisk the oil, lemon juice, garlic and sumac or cumin together in a bowl. Season to taste with salt and pepper.
2. To make the salad, combine the pitta pieces, tomatoes, cucumber, radishes, onion, lettuce leaves and mint leaves in a large bowl.
3. Pour the dressing over the salad and gently mix together to coat the salad evenly.

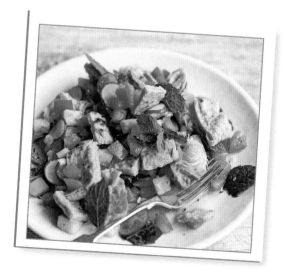

greek salad with toasted pitta

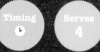

Cost £

Timing 🕐

Serves 4

what you need

- 100 g (3½ oz) feta cheese, crumbled into smallish chunks
- 8–10 fresh mint leaves, shredded
- 100 g (3½ oz) kalamata olives, pitted
- 2 tomatoes, chopped
- juice of 1 large lemon
- 1 small red onion, thinly sliced
- 1 teaspoon dried oregano
- 4 pitta breads
- lemon wedges, to serve

what you do

1. Put the feta, mint, olives, tomatoes, lemon juice, onion and oregano in a bowl and toss together to mix.
2. Toast the pitta breads under a preheated hot grill until lightly golden, turning once, then split open and toast the open sides.
3. Tear the hot pittas into bite-sized pieces, then toss with the other ingredients in the bowl. Serve immediately with lemon wedges.

HEALTHY TIP

Switch regular fizzy drinks for low-calorie versions. Carbonated drinks aren't exactly a healthy addition to your diet but if you're going to treat yourself, at least make it sugar-free.

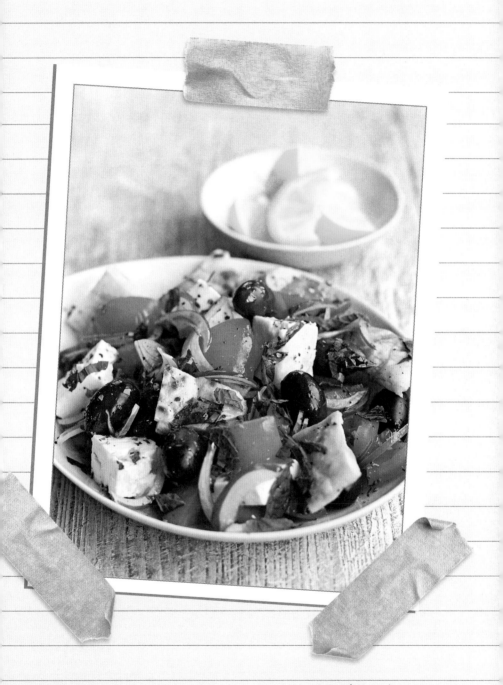

smoked mackerel superfood salad

Cost
££

Timing

Serves
4

- 500 g (1 lb) butternut squash, peeled, deseeded and cut into 1 cm (½ inch) cubes
- 4 tablespoons olive oil
- 1 teaspoon cumin seeds
- 1 head of broccoli, cut into florets
- 200 g (7 oz) frozen or fresh peas
- 3 tablespoons quinoa, rinsed and drained
- 4 tablespoons mixed seeds

- 2 smoked mackerel fillets
- juice of 1 lemon
- 1 teaspoon clear honey
- 1 Dijon mustard
- 100 g (3½ oz) red cabbage, shredded
- 4 tomatoes, chopped
- 4 cooked beetroot, cut into wedges
- 20 g (¾ oz) radish sprouts

what you do

1. Place the squash in a roasting tin and sprinkle with 1 tablespoon of the oil and the cumin seeds. Place in a preheated oven, 200°C (400°F), Gas Mark 6, for 15–18 minutes until tender. Leave to cool slightly.

2. Meanwhile, cook the broccoli in a saucepan of boiling water for 4–5 minutes until tender, adding the frozen peas 3 minutes before the end of the cooking time (4 minutes for fresh peas). Remove with a slotted spoon and refresh under cold running water, then drain (reserving the cooking water). Cook the quinoa in the broccoli water for 15 minutes, then drain and leave to cool slightly.

3. Heat a nonstick frying pan over a medium-low heat and dry-fry the seeds, stirring frequently, until golden brown and toasted. Set aside. Heat the mackerel fillets according to the packet instructions, then skin and break into flakes.

4. Whisk together the remaining oil, the lemon juice, honey and mustard in a small bowl. Toss together all the ingredients, except the radish sprouts, with the dressing in a serving bowl. Serve topped with the radish sprouts.

courgette, feta & mint salad

ost
£

Timing

Serves
1

at you need

- green courgettes
- yellow courgettes
- ive oil, for drizzling
- nall bunch of mint leaves
- 0 g (1½ oz) feta cheese
- alt and pepper

ssing
- tablespoons olive oil
- nely grated rind and juice of
- lemon

1. Thinly slice the courgettes lengthways into long ribbons. Drizzle with oil and season with salt and pepper. Heat a griddle pan until it's very hot, then grill the courgettes, in batches, until tender and griddle-marked on both sides. Transfer to a large salad bowl.
2. Make the dressing by whisking together the oil and lemon rind and juice in a small bowl. Season to taste with salt and pepper.
3. Roughly chop the mint, reserving some leaves for the garnish. Carefully mix together the griddled courgettes, chopped mint and dressing in the salad bowl, then crumble the feta over the top, garnish with the remaining mint leaves and serve.

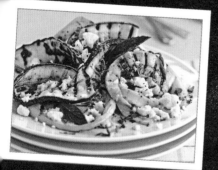

brainfood bowl

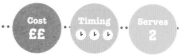

- 100 g (3½ oz) brown rice
- 150 g (5 oz) broccoli florets
- 75 g (3 oz) sugar snap peas, halved lengthways
- 50 g (2 oz) hazelnuts, roughly chopped
- 25 g (1 oz) pumpkin seeds

- 1 pink or red grapefruit
- 1 ripe avocado
- 25 g (1 oz) fresh root ginger, peeled and grated
- 1 tablespoon olive oil
- 1 tablespoon clear honey
- salt and pepper

what you do

1. Cook the rice in a large saucepan of lightly salted water for 25 minutes or until just tender.
2. Meanwhile, cut the broccoli into smaller pieces and cook in a separate saucepan of boiling water for 2 minutes until softened. Add the sugar snap peas and cook for a further 30 seconds. Drain, rinse under cold running water, then drain again.
3. Lightly toast the hazelnuts in a dry frying pan, shaking the pan frequently until the nuts start to colour. Add the pumpkin seeds and cook for a further 1–2 minutes until they start to pop.
4. Thoroughly drain the rice and mix in a bowl with the broccoli, sugar snap peas, nuts and seeds.
5. Halve the grapefruit. Squeeze the juice from one half into a small bowl. Cut away the skin and white pith from the remaining half and chop the flesh. Add to the rice bowl. Peel, halve, stone and dice the avocado and add to the grapefruit juice. Toss to coat, then lift out with a slotted spoon and add to the rice.
6. Whisk the ginger, oil and honey into the grapefruit juice. Stir the dressing into the rice mixture just before serving. Season to taste with salt and pepper and serve.

soy tofu salad with coriander

Cost
£

Timing
🕐

Serves
4

what you need

- 500 g (1 lb) firm tofu, drained
- 6 spring onions, finely shredded
- large handful of fresh coriander leaves, roughly chopped
- 1 large mild red chilli, deseeded and thinly sliced
- 4 tablespoons light soy sauce
- 2 teaspoons sesame oil

what you do

1. Cut the tofu into bite-sized cubes and carefully arrange on a serving plate in a single layer. Sprinkle over the spring onions, coriander and chilli.
2. Drizzle over the soy sauce and oil, then leave to stand at room temperature for 10 minutes before serving.

Variation
For steamed chilli-soy tofu, drain 500 g (1 lb) firm tofu, cut it into bite-sized cubes and place it on a heatproof plate that will fit inside a bamboo steamer. Cover and steam over a wok or large saucepan of boiling water for 20 minutes, then drain off the excess water and carefully transfer to a serving plate. Heat 4 tablespoons light soy sauce, 1 tablespoon each sesame oil and groundnut oil and 2 teaspoons oyster sauce in a small saucepan until hot. Pour over the tofu, scatter with 4 thinly sliced spring onions, 1 finely chopped red chilli and a small handful of finely chopped fresh coriander leaves and serve.

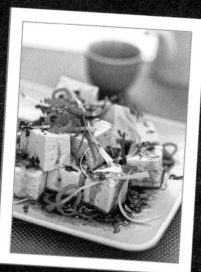

spiced chicken & mango salad

what you need

- 6 teaspoons mild curry paste
- juice of 1 lemon
- 4 small boneless, skinless chicken breasts, cut into long, thin strips
- 150 g (5 oz) natural yogurt
- 1 ripe mango, peeled, stoned and cut into bite-sized chunks
- 50 g (2 oz) watercress, torn into smaller pieces
- ½ cucumber, diced
- ½ red onion, chopped
- ½ iceberg lettuce

what you do

1. Put 4 teaspoons of the curry paste into a polythene food bag with the lemon juice and mix together by squeezing the bag. Add the chicken strips and toss together.
2. Half-fill the base of a steamer with water and bring to the boil. Remove the chicken from the bag and place in the top of the steamer in a single layer. Cover and steam for 5–6 minutes until cooked through.
3. Meanwhile, mix the remaining curry paste in a bowl with the yogurt. Put the mango, watercress, cucumber and onion in a bowl, add the yogurt dressing and toss together gently.
4. Tear the lettuce into pieces, divide it between 4 plates, then spoon the mango mixture on top. Add the warm chicken strips on top, then serve.

Variation

For coronation chicken, mix the curry paste and yogurt with 4 tablespoons reduced-fat mayonnaise. Stir in 500 g (1 lb) cold cooked diced chicken and 40 g (1½ oz) sultanas. Sprinkle with 25 g (1 oz) toasted flaked almonds and serve on a bed of mixed salad and herb leaves.

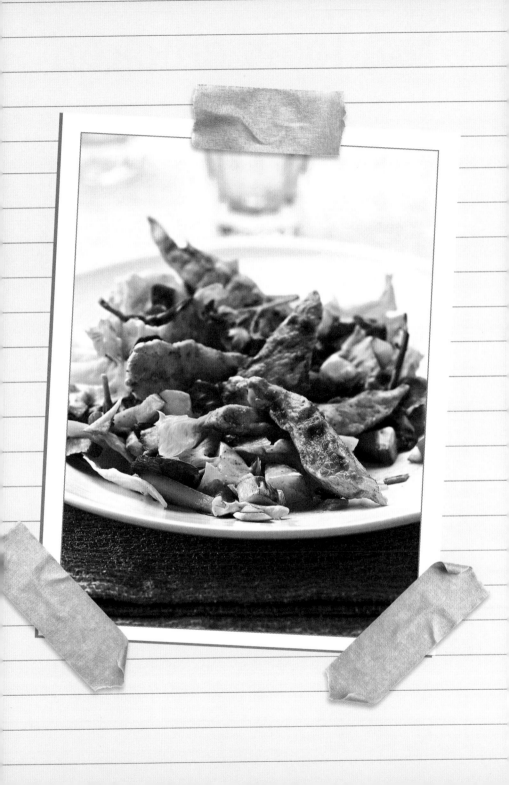

tandoori chicken salad

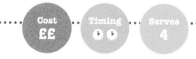

Cost
££

Timing
▷ ▷

Serves
4

- 200 ml (7 fl oz) natural yogurt
- 2 tablespoons lemon juice
- ½ teaspoon ground turmeric
- 1 teaspoon garam masala
- 1 teaspoon cumin seeds, roughly crushed
- 2 tablespoons tomato purée
- 2 garlic cloves, finely chopped
- 1.5 cm (¾ inch) piece of fresh root ginger, peeled and finely chopped

- 3 boneless, skinless chicken breasts, thickly sliced
- 1 tablespoon sunflower oil

Salad
- 200 g (7 oz) mixed salad leaves
- small bunch of fresh coriander
- 4 tablespoons lemon juice

what You do

1. Mix the yogurt, lemon juice, spices, tomato purée, garlic and ginger together in a shallow, non-metallic dish. Add the chicken and toss to coat. Cover and leave to marinate in the fridge for 3–4 hours or until required.
2. When you are ready to serve, heat the oil in a large frying pan. Lift the chicken out of the marinade and add to the pan. Cook over a medium heat for 8–10 minutes, turning occasionally, until the chicken is browned and cooked through.
3. Meanwhile, for the salad, toss the salad leaves, coriander and lemon juice together in a bowl and then divide between serving plates. Spoon the hot chicken on top and serve immediately.

turkey & avocado salad

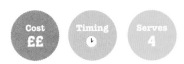

Cost
££

Timing
◔

Serves
4

what you need

- 1 large ripe avocado, peeled, stoned and diced
- 1 punnet of mustard and cress, cut
- 150 g (5 oz) mixed salad leaves
- 375 g (12 oz) cooked turkey, thinly sliced
- 50 g (2 oz) mixed toasted seeds, such as pumpkin and sunflower
- toasted wholegrain rye bread or flatbreads, to serve

Dressing
- 2 tablespoons apple juice
- 2 tablespoons natural yogurt
- 1 teaspoon clear honey
- 1 teaspoon wholegrain mustard
- salt and pepper

1. Put the avocado, mustard and cress and salad leaves in a large bowl and mix together. Add the turkey and toasted seeds and stir to combine.
2. Make the dressing by whisking together the apple juice, yogurt, honey and mustard in a small bowl. Season to taste with salt and pepper.
3. Pour the dressing over the salad and toss to mix. Serve the salad with toasted wholegrain rye bread or rolled up in flatbreads.

Variation
For a crab, apple and avocado salad, prepare the salad in the same way, using 300 g (10 oz) cooked, fresh white crab meat instead of the turkey. Cut 1 peeled and cored dessert apple into thin matchsticks and toss with a little lemon juice to stop it from discolouring. Add to the crab salad. Make a dressing by whisking together 2 tablespoons apple juice, 3 tablespoons olive oil, a squeeze of lemon juice and 1 finely diced shallot. Season to taste with salt and pepper. Pour the dressing over the salad, stir carefully to mix and serve.

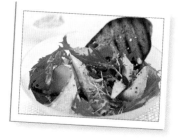

tuna & borlotti bean salad

what you need

Cost £
Timing ●
Serves 4

- 400 g (13 oz) can borlotti beans, rinsed and drained
- 1 tablespoon water (optional)
- 2 tablespoons extra virgin olive oil
- 2 garlic cloves, crushed
- 1 red chilli, deseeded and finely chopped
- 2 celery sticks, thinly sliced

- 1½ red onions, cut into thin wedges
- 200 g (7 oz) can tuna in olive oil, drained and flaked
- finely grated rind and juice of 1 lemon
- 50 g (2 oz) rocket leaves
- salt and pepper

what you do

1. Heat the borlotti beans in a saucepan over a medium heat for 3 minutes, adding the water if the beans start to stick to the base.
2. Put the oil, garlic and chilli in a large bowl. Stir in the celery, onions and hot beans and season with salt and pepper. Cover and leave to marinate at room temperature for at least 30 minutes and up to 4 hours.
3. Stir in the tuna and lemon rind and juice. Gently toss in the rocket, taste and adjust the seasoning with extra salt, pepper and lemon juice, if necessary, then serve.

Variation

For a mixed bean salad, heat the borlotti beans, as above, with a 400 g (13 oz) can rinsed and drained cannellini beans. Leave to marinate with the other salad ingredients as above, but also adding 2 tablespoons roughly chopped flat leaf parsley. After marinating, toss in 50 g (2 oz) lamb's lettuce, season with salt and pepper and serve.

crab &
grapefruit salad

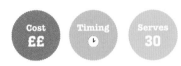

Cost	Timing	Serves
££	🕐	30

what you do

what you need

- 400 g (13 oz) white crab meat
- 1 pink grapefruit, peeled, white pith removed and flesh sliced
- 50 g (2 oz) rocket
- 3 spring onions, sliced
- 200 g (7 oz) mangetout, halved
- salt and pepper

Watercress dressing
- 90 g (3¼ oz) watercress (tough stalks removed), chopped
- 1 tablespoon Dijon mustard
- 2 tablespoons olive oil

To serve
- 4 chapattis
- lime wedges

1. Combine the crab meat, grapefruit, rocket, spring onions and mangetout in a serving dish. Season to taste with salt and pepper.
2. Make the dressing by whisking together the watercress, mustard and oil in a small bowl. Season to taste with salt.
3. Toast the chapattis. Stir the dressing into the crab salad, then serve with the toasted chapattis and lime wedges on the side.

Variation
For a prawn, potato and asparagus salad, substitute 400 g (13 oz) cooked peeled prawns for the crab and 100 g (3½ oz) cooked asparagus for the grapefruit, and add 200 g (7 oz) cooked and cooled potatoes.

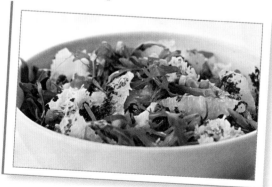

quick one-pot ratatouille

Cost
£

Timing
⏱ ⏱

Serves
4

what you need

- 100 ml (3½ fl oz) olive oil
- 2 onions, chopped
- 1 aubergine, cut into bite-sized cubes
- 2 large courgettes, cut into bite-sized pieces
- 1 red pepper, cored, deseeded and cut into bite-sized pieces
- 1 yellow pepper, cored, deseeded and cut into bite-sized pieces
- 2 garlic cloves, crushed
- 400 g (13 oz) can chopped tomatoes
- 4 tablespoons chopped parsley or basil
- salt and pepper

what you do

1. Heat the oil in a large saucepan until very hot. Add the onions, aubergine, courgettes, peppers and garlic and cook, stirring constantly, for a few minutes until softened.
2. Add the tomatoes, season with salt and pepper and stir well. Reduce the heat, cover the pan tightly and simmer for 15 minutes until all the vegetables are cooked. Remove from the heat and stir in the parsley or basil before serving.

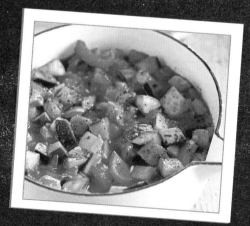

goats' cheese & spinach quesadillas

Cost
££

Timing

Serves
4

what you do

what you need

- 275 g (9 oz) baby spinach leaves
- 8 soft flour tortillas
- 250 g (8 oz) goats' cheese
- 2 tablespoons drained, chopped sun-dried tomatoes
- 2 ripe avocados, peeled, stoned and diced
- 1 red onion, thinly sliced
- juice of 1 lime
- 2 tablespoons chopped fresh coriander
- salt and pepper

1. Place the spinach in a saucepan with a small amount of water, then cover and cook until wilted. Drain and squeeze dry.
2. Heat a nonstick frying pan over medium heat until hot, add 1 tortilla and then crumble a quarter of the goats' cheese, followed by a quarter of the spinach and sun-dried tomatoes, over the tortilla. Season lightly with salt and pepper.
3. Place 1 tortilla on top and cook for 3–4 minutes until golden underneath. Carefully turn the quesadilla over and cook for a further 3–4 minutes. Remove from the pan and keep warm. Repeat with the remaining 6 tortillas.
4. Meanwhile, mix together the avocados, onion, lime juice and coriander in a bowl.
5. Serve the warm quesadillas cut into wedges with the avocado salsa.

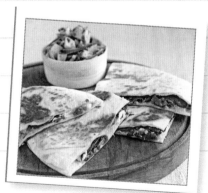

smoked mackerel & chive pâté

Cost
£

Timing

Serves
8

what you need

- 200 g (7 oz) smoked mackerel, skinned, boned and flaked
- 125 g (4 oz) low-fat soft cheese
- bunch of chives, snipped
- 1 tablespoon fat-free vinaigrette
- 1 tablespoon lemon juice
- vegetable crudités and wholemeal toast, to serve (optional)

HEALTHY TIP

Of all the oily fish that are readily available, mackerel is the richest source of omega-3 fatty acids, so enjoy it in all its many forms — fresh, canned or smoked. It is also one of the least expensive oily fish.

what you do

1. Place the mackerel and soft cheese in a bowl and mash together. Add all the remaining ingredients and mix well. Alternatively, mix all the ingredients together in a blender or food processor.
2. Spoon the mixture into 8 small individual serving dishes or 1 large serving dish. Cover and refrigerate for at least 2 hours or up to 4 hours, before serving.
3. Serve the mackerel pâté with vegetable crudités and wholemeal toast, if liked.

Variation

Try using other omega-3-rich fish instead of mackerel in this recipe, such as canned (in water) drained pilchards, salmon or tuna.

hot & smoky hummus with warm flatbread

Cost
£

Timing
◔

Serves
4

what you need

- 400 g (13 oz) can chickpeas, rinsed and drained
- 3 tablespoons lemon juice
- 1 large garlic clove, crushed
- 2 tablespoons tahini
- 1 teaspoon hot smoked paprika, plus extra for sprinkling
- ½ teaspoon ground cumin
- 150 ml (¼ pint) extra virgin olive oil, plus extra for drizzling
- 2 tablespoons sesame seeds
- salt and pepper

To serve
- 4 Lebanese or Turkish flatbreads
- crunchy raw vegetable crudités (optional)

what you do

1. Put all the ingredients, except the olive oil, sesame seeds and salt and pepper in a blender or food processor and process until smooth. With the machine still running, very slowly drizzle the oil into the chickpea paste until it is all completely incorporated. Season to taste with salt and pepper and then scrape the hummus into a small dish.

2. Heat a dry, nonstick frying pan and toast the sesame seeds over a medium-low heat, moving them quickly around the pan until they are golden brown. Stir most of the sesame seeds into the hummus, then sprinkle the rest over the top.

3. Wrap the flatbreads in foil and heat in a preheated oven, 160°C (325°F), Gas Mark 3, for about 10 minutes until warmed through. Drizzle the hummus with olive oil, sprinkle with smoked paprika and serve with the warm flatbreads and crunchy vegetable crudités, if liked.

guacamole

Cost £

Timing ⏱

Serves 4

what you need

- 2 ripe avocados, peeled, stoned and chopped
- juice of 1 lime
- 6 cherry tomatoes, diced
- 1 tablespoon chopped fresh coriander
- 1-2 garlic cloves, crushed
- oatcakes or vegetable crudités, to serve

what you do

1. Put the avocados and lime juice in a bowl and mash together to prevent discoloration, then stir in the remaining ingredients.
2. Serve immediately with oatcakes or vegetable crudités.

HEALTHY TIP

Download a pedometer.
There are plenty of free pedometer apps available and this is a great way to check your daily activity. Aim for 10,000 steps a day to help maintain a healthy lifestyle.

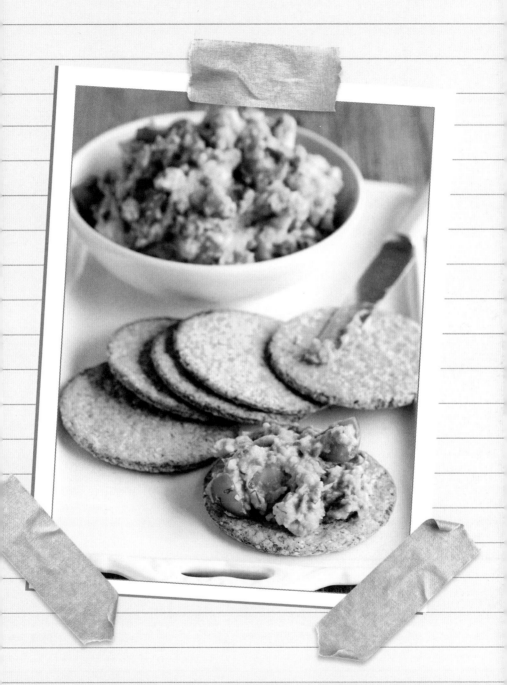

spicy courgette fritters

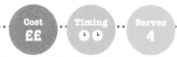

Cost ££ **Timing** ▶ ▶ **Serves** 4

what you need

- 3 courgettes
- 2 large spring onions, grated or very finely chopped
- 1 garlic clove, finely chopped
- finely grated rind of 1 lemon
- 4 tablespoons gram flour
- 2 teaspoons medium curry powder
- 1 red chilli, deseeded and finely chopped

- 2 tablespoons finely chopped mint leaves
- 2 tablespoons finely chopped fresh coriander leaves
- 2 eggs, lightly beaten
- 2 tablespoons light olive oil
- salt and pepper

what you do

1. Grate the courgettes into a colander. Sprinkle lightly with salt and leave for at least 1 hour to drain. Squeeze out the remaining liquid.
2. Place the remaining ingredients, except the eggs and oil, in a mixing bowl and add the grated courgettes. Season lightly with salt and pepper, bearing in mind you have already salted the courgettes, and mix well. Add the eggs and mix again to combine.
3. Heat half of the oil in a large frying pan over a medium-high heat. Place dessertspoonfuls of the mixture (in batches), well spaced, in the pan and press down with the back of the spoon. Cook for 1–2 minutes on each side, until golden and cooked through. Remove from the pan and keep warm. Repeat to cook the rest of the fritters in the same way, adding the remaining oil to the pan when necessary. Serve warm.

salmon & rice bhajis

what you need

Cost
££

Timing
🕐 🕐

Serves
4

- 2 x 170 g (6 oz) cans salmon, drained and flaked
- 1 small onion, sliced
- ½ teaspoon ground cumin
- ¼ teaspoon dried chilli flakes
- 2 tablespoons chopped fresh coriander
- 75 g (3 oz) cooked cold white rice (see page 167)
- 1 egg, beaten
- 1–2 tablespoons plain flour
- 2 tablespoons rapeseed oil
- 150 ml (¼ pint) natural yogurt
- ½ cucumber, grated
- 1 tablespoon chopped mint
- salt and pepper

what you do

1. Place the salmon, onion, spices, coriander and rice in a large bowl and mix well. Stir in the egg and season well with salt and pepper. Mix in enough of the flour to form a stiff mixture. Using wet hands, shape into 20 small balls.
2. Heat the oil in a large frying pan, add the bhajis and fry for 3–4 minutes, turning once, until golden.
3. Meanwhile, mix together the yogurt, cucumber and mint in a bowl. Serve with the hot bhajis.

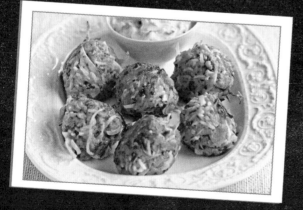

light egg-fried rice

 Cost £

 Timing ⏱

 Serves 4

what you do

what you need

- 4 eggs
- 2 teaspoons peeled and finely chopped fresh root ginger
- 1½ tablespoons light soy sauce
- 2 tablespoons groundnut oil
- 300 g (10 oz) freshly cooked jasmine rice or long-grain rice (see page 167), cooled
- 2 spring onions, thinly sliced
- ¼ teaspoon sesame oil

1. Beat the eggs with the ginger and half of the soy sauce in a bowl until combined.
2. Heat the groundnut oil in a nonstick wok or large frying pan over a high heat until the oil starts to shimmer. Pour in the egg mixture and cook, stirring constantly, for 30 seconds or until softly scrambled.
3. Add the cooked rice, spring onions, sesame oil and remaining soy sauce to the pan and toss together for about 1–2 minutes until the rice is piping hot. Serve immediately.

Variation
For fried rice with Chinese leaves and chilli, follow the recipe above, adding 1 deseeded and sliced red chilli and 125 g (4 oz) shredded Chinese leaves once the rice is piping hot, tossing together for a further 30 seconds.

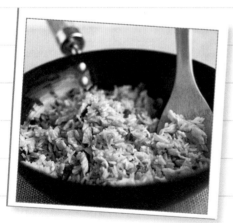

chilli kale

what you need

- 1 tablespoon olive oil
- 1 garlic clove, crushed
- 1 large onion, chopped
- 500 g (1 lb) curly kale, stalks removed and leaves chopped
- 2 teaspoons lime juice
- 1 red chilli, deseeded and chopped
- salt and pepper

what you do

1. Heat the oil in a wok or large frying pan over a medium heat. Add the garlic and onion and stir-fry for 5–10 minutes or until the onion is translucent.
2. Add the curly kale and stir-fry for a further 5 minutes. Stir in the lime juice and chilli, season with salt and pepper to taste and then serve immediately.

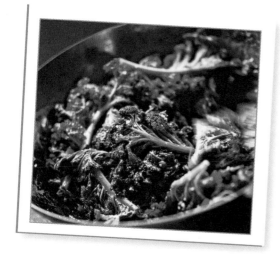

Variation
For chilli cabbage, replace the curly kale with 500 g (1 lb) cabbage. Discard the stalks and tough outer leaves, then chop the leaves before frying with the softened garlic and onion, then finishing as above. This recipe also works well with spring greens.

quick spinach with pine nuts

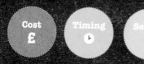

Cost
£

Timing
🕐

Serves
4

what you need

- 1 tablespoon olive oil
- 1 red onion, sliced
- 1 garlic clove, crushed
- 75 g (3 oz) pine nuts
- 4 tomatoes, skinned, cored and roughly chopped
- 1 kg (2 lb) spinach, washed and trimmed
- 50 g (2 oz) butter
- pinch of freshly grated nutmeg
- salt and pepper

what you do

1. Heat the oil in a large saucepan, add the onion and garlic and sauté for 5 minutes.
2. Put the pine nuts into a small, heavy-based frying pan and dry-fry until browned, stirring constantly as they turn brown very quickly. Remove from the heat.
3. Add the tomatoes, spinach, butter and nutmeg to the onion and garlic and season with salt and pepper. Turn up the heat to high and mix well. Cook for 3 minutes until the spinach has just started to wilt, stirring frequently.
4. Remove from the heat, stir in the pine nuts and serve immediately.

potato wedges with yogurt & parsley dip

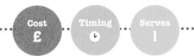

what you do

1. Cut the potato into 8 wedges and cook them in a saucepan of lightly salted boiling water for 5 minutes. Drain the wedges thoroughly, then put them into a bowl with the red pepper slices and toss with the oil. Sprinkle with paprika and salt to taste.

2. Arrange the potato wedges and pepper slices on a baking tray and cook under a preheated hot grill for 6–8 minutes, turning occasionally, until cooked.

3. Meanwhile, for the yogurt and parsley dip, put the yogurt, parsley, spring onions and garlic, if using, into a bowl. Season to taste with salt and pepper and mix thoroughly.

4. Serve the potato wedges and pepper slices hot with the yogurt dip.

what you need

- 1 potato, about 175 g (6 oz)
- 1 red pepper, cored, deseeded and sliced
- 1 teaspoon olive oil
- paprika, to taste
- salt and pepper

Yogurt and parsley dip
- 3 tablespoons natural yogurt
- 1 tablespoon chopped parsley
- 2 spring onions, chopped
- 1 garlic clove, crushed (optional)

healthy
mashed potatoes

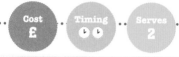

Cost
£

Timing
◑ ◑

Serves
2

what you need

- 500 g (1 lb) floury potatoes
- 50 ml (2 fl oz) half-fat crème fraîche
- salt and pepper

what you do

1. Cut the potatoes into chunks and cook in a large saucepan of lightly salted, boiling water for 15–20 minutes until tender. Drain, reserving 2 tablespoons of the cooking water and return the potatoes to the saucepan with the water.
2. Mash well until smooth. Stir in the crème fraîche and plenty of pepper, then serve.

Variations

Mix and match any of the following ingredients, adding when mashing: finely grated rind of 1 lemon; a handful of finely chopped herbs such as dill, parsley, chervil, tarragon or chives; 2 tablespoons chopped (drained) capers or a small garlic clove, finely crushed. You can also use 3–4 tablespoons olive oil or milk instead of the crème fraîche, or swap half of the potatoes for the same weight of parsnips, celeriac or carrots, cooking them in the same pan as the potatoes.

courgette & ricotta bakes

what you need

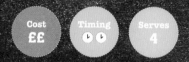

Cost
££

Timing
⏱ ⏱

Serves
4

- butter, for greasing
- 2 courgettes
- 100 g (3½ oz) fresh white or wholemeal breadcrumbs
- 250 g (8 oz) ricotta cheese
- 75 g (3 oz) Parmesan-style cheese, grated
- 2 eggs, beaten
- 1 garlic clove, crushed
- handful of chopped basil
- salt and pepper

Variation

For mushrooms stuffed with courgettes and ricotta, brush a little olive oil over 4 large field mushrooms, trimmed, and place on a baking tray, stalk side up. Grate 1 courgette and squeeze to remove any excess moisture, then mix with 200 g (7 oz) ricotta cheese, 4 drained and chopped sun-dried tomatoes in oil and 25 g (1 oz) chopped pitted black olives. Season with salt and pepper, spoon on to the mushrooms, then sprinkle with 25 g (1 oz) grated Parmesan-style cheese. Bake in a preheated oven, 200°C (400°F), Gas Mark 6, for 15 minutes until golden and cooked through. Serve with ciabatta rolls.

what you do

1. Grease 8 holes of a muffin tin.
2. Use a vegetable peeler to make 16 long ribbons of courgette and set aside. Coarsely grate the remaining courgettes and squeeze to remove any excess moisture. Mix the grated courgettes with all the remaining ingredients in a bowl and season well with salt and pepper.
3. Arrange 2 courgette ribbons in a cross shape in each hole of the prepared muffin tin. Spoon in the filling and then fold over the overhanging courgette ends. Bake in a preheated oven, 190°C (375°F), Gas Mark 5, for 15–20 minutes or until golden and cooked through. Turn out on to serving plates and serve immediately.

Sweet Alternatives

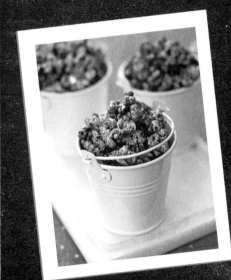

strawberry & almond layered desserts

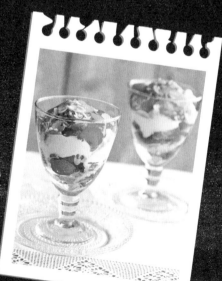

toffee & chocolate popcorn

courgette, lemon & poppy seed cake ....

blackcurrant polenta mug cake ....

spiced passion mug cake ....

gluten-free coconut & mango cake ....

chocolate, courgette & nut cake ....

lemon drizzle cake ....

easy almond macaroons ....

chocolate peanut cookies ....

cranberry & hazelnut cookies ....

toffee & chocolate popcorn ....

mango & passion fruit trifle ....

baked strawberries & meringue ....

roasted honey peaches ....

berry & mint compote ....

instant apple crumbles ....

strawberry & almond layered desserts ....

lemon & sultana rice pudding ....

warm chocolate fromage frais ....

white chocolate mousse ....

cidered apple jellies ....

griddled bananas with blueberries ....

courgette, lemon & poppy seed cake

Cost
££

Timing

Serves
8

what you need

- 75 ml (3 fl oz) olive oil, plus extra for greasing
- 150 g (5 oz) spelt flour
- 1 teaspoon baking powder
- 2 eggs
- 50 ml (2 fl oz) clear honey
- 50 g (2 oz) caster sugar
- 2 tablespoons poppy seeds
- finely grated rind and juice of 1 lemon
- 100 g (3½ oz) courgette, grated

Frosting
- 125 ml (4 fl oz) 0%-fat Greek yogurt
- 2 tablespoons lemon curd

what you do

1. Grease and line with greaseproof paper a loaf tin with a capacity of about 500 g (1 lb).
2. Sift the flour and baking powder into a bowl. Beat the eggs in a separate mixing bowl with the oil, honey, sugar, poppy seeds and lemon rind and juice. Stir in the grated courgette. Add the flour and stir gently to mix.
3. Transfer the mixture to the prepared tin and level the surface. Bake in a preheated oven 160°C (325°F), Gas Mark 3, for 40–45 minutes or until risen and just firm to the touch. A skewer inserted into the centre should come out clean. Transfer to a wire rack to cool.
4. For the frosting, spoon the yogurt on to several sheets of kitchen paper. Place several more sheets on top and press firmly to squeeze out as much liquid as possible. Turn the yogurt into a bowl and stir in the lemon curd. Spread over the top of the cold cake. Serve in slices.

blackcurrant polenta mug cake

Cost
£

Timing
◐

Serves
1

- 2 tablespoons polenta
- 25 g (1 oz) slightly salted butter, softened
- 2 tablespoons clear honey, plus extra to drizzle
- 2 tablespoons ground almonds
- 1 egg
- 2 tablespoons blackcurrants, topped and tailed
- 1 tablespoon blackcurrant preserve

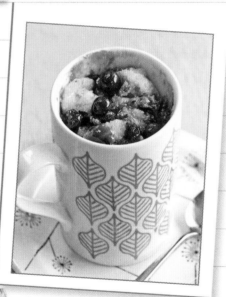

what you do

1. Beat together the polenta, butter, honey and ground almonds in a 200 ml (7 fl oz) microwave-proof mug. Add the egg and beat together until well mixed. Microwave on full power for 1 minute.
2. Spoon the blackcurrants and blackcurrant preserve on top and stir in lightly so the polenta mixture is marbled with the fruit. Microwave on full power for 1 minute. Serve drizzled with extra honey.

spiced passion mug cake

Cost
££

Timing

Serves
1

what You do

1. Put the honey, butter, egg, flour and ginger in a 350 ml (12 fl oz) microwave-proof mug and beat together until well mixed. Add the carrot and pineapple and mix thoroughly.
2. Microwave on full power for 2 minutes or until just firm to touch and a cocktail stick inserted into the centre comes out clean. Serve the cake topped with the cream cheese and drizzled with the ginger syrup.

what You need

- 2 tablespoons clear honey
- 25 g (1 oz) slightly salted butter, softened
- 1 egg
- 3 tablespoons self-raising flour
- 2.5 cm (1 inch) piece of preserved stem ginger in syrup, drained and chopped
- 5 cm (2 inch) piece of carrot, finely grated
- ½ fresh or canned pineapple ring, chopped
- 1 tablespoon cream cheese
- 1 tablespoon preserved stem ginger syrup, to drizzle

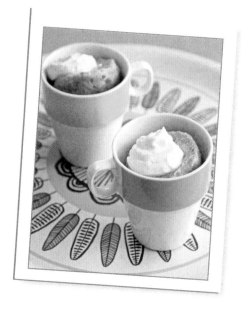

gluten-free coconut & mango cake

Cost
£££

Timing

Serves
12

what you need

- 100 g (3½ oz) butter, softened, plus extra for greasing
- 100 g (3½ oz) soft light brown sugar
- 4 eggs, separated
- 400 ml (14 fl oz) buttermilk
- 200 g (7 oz) polenta
- 200 g (7 oz) rice flour
- 2 teaspoons gluten-free baking powder
- 50 g (2 oz) coconut milk powder
- 50 g (2 oz) desiccated coconut
- 1 ripe mango, peeled, stoned and flesh puréed

Filling
- 250 g (8 oz) mascarpone cheese
- 1 ripe mango, peeled, stoned and finely chopped
- 2 tablespoons icing sugar

what you do

1. Grease and line with greaseproof paper a 23 cm (9 inch) round, deep, loose-bottomed cake tin.
2. Place the butter and brown sugar in a large bowl and beat together until light and fluffy, then beat in the egg yolks, buttermilk, polenta, rice flour, baking powder, coconut milk powder and desiccated coconut. Whisk the egg whites in a separate large, clean bowl until they form soft peaks, then fold into the cake mixture with the puréed mango.
3. Spoon the mixture into the prepared tin, level the surface, then bake in a preheated oven, 200°C (400°F) Gas Mark 6, for 45-50 minutes until golden and firm to the touch. Let cool in the tin for 5 minutes. Transfer to a wire rack to cool completely.
4. When the cake is cold, slice it in half horizontally. Place the filling ingredients in a bowl and mix together until combined. Use half of the filling to sandwich the cake together, then spread the remaining mixture over the top. Serve in slices.

chocolate, courgette & nut cake

- 100 ml (3½ fl oz) vegetable oil, plus extra for greasing
- 250 g (8 oz) courgettes, coarsely grated
- 2 eggs
- finely grated rind and juice of 1 orange
- 125 g (4 oz) caster sugar
- 225 g (7½ oz) self-raising flour
- 2 tablespoons cocoa powder
- ½ teaspoon bicarbonate of soda
- ½ teaspoon baking powder
- 50 g (2 oz) ready-to-eat dried apricots, chopped

Topping
- 200 g (7 oz) cream cheese
- 2 tablespoons vegetarian-friendly chocolate hazelnut spread
- 1 tablespoon hazelnuts, toasted and chopped

what you do

1. Grease and line with greaseproof paper a 20 cm (8 inch) round, deep, loose-bottomed cake tin.
2. Place the courgettes in a sieve and squeeze out any excess liquid. Beat together the eggs, oil, orange rind and juice and sugar in a large bowl. Sift in the flour, cocoa powder, bicarbonate of soda and baking powder and beat to combine. Fold in the courgettes and apricots, then spoon the mixture into the prepared tin and level the surface.
3. Bake in a preheated oven, 180°C (350°F), Gas Mark 4, for 40 minutes until risen and firm to the touch. Let cool in the tin for 5 minutes. Turn out on to a wire rack and leave to cool completely.
4. For the topping, beat together the cream cheese and chocolate hazelnut spread in a bowl, then spread over the top of the cake. Sprinkle over the chopped hazelnuts. Serve in slices.

lemon drizzle cake

what you need

Cost £ · **Timing** · **Serves** 8

- 100 g (3½ oz) butter, melted and cooled, plus extra for greasing
- 5 eggs
- 100 g (3½ oz) caster sugar
- pinch of salt
- 125 g (4 oz) plain flour
- 1 teaspoon baking powder
- finely grated rind of 1 lemon
- 1 tablespoon lemon juice

Syrup
- 250 g (8 oz) icing sugar, sifted
- 125 ml (4 fl oz) lemon juice
- finely grated rind of 1 lemon
- seeds scraped from 1 vanilla pod

- half-fat crème fraîche or low-fat soured cream, to serve

what you do

1. Grease and line with greaseproof paper a 22 cm (8½ inch) square cake tin.
2. Put the eggs, caster sugar and salt in a large, heatproof bowl set over a saucepan of barely simmering water and beat with a hand-held electric whisk for 2-3 minutes or until the mixture triples in volume and thickens to the consistency of lightly whipped cream. Remove from the heat. Sift in the flour and baking powder, add the grated lemon rind and juice and drizzle the butter down the side of the bowl. Fold in gently.
3. Pour the mixture into the prepared tin. Bake in a preheated oven, 180°C (350°F), Gas Mark 4, for 20-25 minutes or until risen, golden and coming away from the sides of the tin.
4. Meanwhile, put all the syrup ingredients in a small saucepan and heat gently until the sugar dissolves, stirring. Increase the heat and boil rapidly, without stirring, for 4-5 minutes. Set aside to cool a little.
5. Leave the cake to cool in the tin for 5 minutes, then make holes over the surface with a skewer. Drizzle over two-thirds of the warm syrup (reserve the rest). Leave the cake to cool completely in the tin and absorb the syrup.
6. Turn the cake out of the tin and peel off the lining paper. Cut into squares or slices and serve each portion with about 1 heaped teaspoon of half-fat crème fraîche or soured cream and an extra drizzle of the remaining syrup.

easy almond macaroons

what you need

Cost £€

Timing ⏱

Serves 6

- 2 egg whites
- 100 g (3½ oz) golden caster sugar
- 100 g (3½ oz) ground almonds
- blanched whole almonds, to decorate

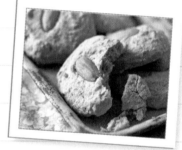

what you do

1. Line a large baking sheet with nonstick baking paper.
2. Whisk the egg whites in a clean bowl with a hand-held electric whisk until soft peaks form. Gradually whisk in the sugar, a spoonful at a time, until thick and glossy. Fold in the ground almonds until combined.
3. Drop dessertspoonfuls of the mixture, slightly apart, on to the prepared baking sheet. Press an almond on top of each.
4. Bake in a preheated oven, 180°C (350°F), Gas Mark 4, for about 15 minutes until the biscuits are pale golden and just crisp. Leave on the paper to cool for 5 minutes, then transfer to a wire rack to cool completely before serving.

Variation

For scribbled chocolate macaroons, make the macaroons as above, replacing 20 g (¾ oz) of the ground almonds with 20 g (¾ oz) cocoa powder and omitting the whole almonds. Heat 50 g (2 oz) plain dark or milk chocolate, evenly chopped, in a microwave-proof mug in a microwave in two or three 30-second bursts, stirring inbetween, until melted. Drizzle over the cooled biscuits with a teaspoon. Leave the chocolate to set before serving.

chocolate peanut cookies

Cost
££

Timing
⏱

Serves
20

what you do

1. Line a large baking sheet with nonstick baking paper.
2. Combine the flour, bicarbonate of soda and sugar in a bowl. Add the peanut butter, honey, oil and chocolate and mix to form a thick paste.
3. Take spoonfuls of the mixture and roll between the palms of your hands into a ball, each about the size of a whole walnut. Space well apart on the prepared baking sheet.
4. Bake in a preheated oven 190°C (375°F), Gas Mark 5, for 10 minutes until the cookies have risen and turned golden. Leave on the baking sheet for 2 minutes to firm up, then transfer to a wire rack to cool completely.

what you need

- 100 g (3½ oz) rice flour
- 1 teaspoon bicarbonate of soda
- 50 g (2 oz) light muscovado sugar
- 200 g (7 oz) crunchy peanut butter
- 50 g (2 oz) clear honey
- 2 tablespoons mild olive oil or vegetable oil
- 75 g (3 oz) plain dark chocolate, chopped

cranberry & hazelnut cookies

what you need

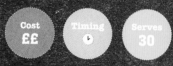

Cost	Timing	Serves
££		30

- 50 g (2 oz) unsalted butter, softened
- 40 g (1½ oz) granulated sugar
- 25 g (1 oz) soft light brown sugar
- 1 egg, beaten
- 1 teaspoon vanilla extract

- 150 g (5 oz) self-raising flour, sifted
- 50 g (2 oz) rolled oats
- 50 g (2 oz) dried cranberries
- 40 g (1½ oz) hazelnuts, toasted and chopped

what you do

1. Line 2 large baking sheets with greaseproof or nonstick baking paper.
2. Beat together the butter, sugars, egg and vanilla extract in a large bowl until smooth. Stir in the flour and oats, then the cranberries and hazelnuts.
3. Place teaspoonfuls of the mixture on to the prepared baking sheets, leaving space between each one, then flatten them slightly with the back of a fork.
4. Bake in a preheated oven, 180°C (350°F), Gas Mark 4, for about 5-6 minutes until lightly browned. Let cool for 2-3 minutes. Transfer to a wire rack and leave to cool completely.

Variation

For plain dark chocolate and ginger cookies, prepare the mixture as above, omitting the dried cranberries and hazelnuts. Replace them with 40 g (1½ oz) plain dark chocolate chips or chunks and 2 pieces of drained, chopped preserved stem ginger (or ½ teaspoon peeled and grated fresh root ginger). Stir together, then bake and cool as above.

toffee & chocolate popcorn

Cost
£

Timing
🕐

Serves
12

what you need

- 125 g (4 oz) popping corn
- 250 g (8 oz) butter
- 250 g (8 oz) light muscovado sugar
- 2 tablespoons cocoa powder

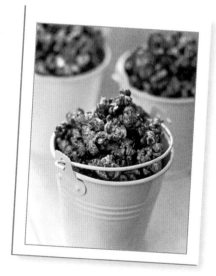

1. Put the popping corn in a large bowl. Cover the bowl with a vented food cover (or greaseproof paper held in place with an elastic band with slits cut into it). Microwave on full power for 4 minutes. Alternatively, cook in a pan with a lid on the hob, over a medium heat, for a few minutes, shaking the pan occasionally to avoid burning the kernels, until popping rapidly then remove from the heat and leave until the popping stops.
2. Meanwhile, gently heat the butter, muscovado sugar and cocoa powder together in a pan, stirring until the sugar has dissolved and the butter has melted. Stir the warm popcorn into the mixture and serve.

Variation

For toffee, marshmallow and nut popcorn, omit the muscovado sugar and cocoa powder. Microwave the popping corn as above, then gently heat 150 g (5 oz) chewy toffees, 125 g (4 oz) butter, 125 g (4 oz) marshmallows and 50 g (2 oz) plain dark chocolate in a pan until melted and combined. Serve as above.

mango & passion fruit trifle

what you need

Cost
££

Timing

Serves
2

- 2 sponge fingers
- 75 ml (3 fl oz) 0%-fat Greek yogurt
- 100 ml (3 ½ fl oz) half-fat crème fraîche
- 2 passion fruit
- ½ ripe mango, peeled, stoned and diced

what you do

1. Break each sponge finger into 4 pieces and divide between 2 glasses. Mix the yogurt and crème fraîche together in a bowl.
2. Halve the passion fruit and scoop out the pulpy seeds. Spoon two-thirds of the seeds over the sponge fingers, then add half of the mango pieces.
3. Spoon half of the crème fraîche mixture over the fruit, then top with the remaining mango. Spoon over the remaining crème fraîche mixture and top with the remaining passion fruit seeds. Chill in the fridge for 1 hour before serving.

baked strawberries & meringue

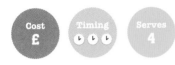

Cost £

Timing

Serves 4

what you need

- 3 egg whites
- 150 g (5 oz) light muscovado sugar
- 1 tablespoon cornflour
- 1 teaspoon white vinegar
- 1 teaspoon vanilla extract
- 250 g (8 oz) strawberries, hulled and sliced

what you do

1. Line 4 individual tart tins or ramekins with nonstick baking paper.
2. Whisk the egg whites in a bowl until they form stiff peaks, then beat in the sugar, a spoonful at a time, making sure the sugar is incorporated between additions. Fold in the cornflour, vinegar and vanilla extract until combined.
3. Spoon the mixture into the prepared tart tins or ramekins and cook in a preheated oven, 120°C (250°F), Gas Mark ½, for 2½ hours. Place the strawberries in an ovenproof dish and bake with the meringues for the last hour of the cooking time.
4. Spoon the baked strawberries and any cooking juices over the meringues to serve.

Variation

For baked nectarines with orange meringues, add the finely grated rind of 1 orange to the meringue mixture with the cornflour. Cut 2 peeled and stoned nectarines into thin slices and place in an ovenproof dish. Sprinkle with 2 tablespoons sugar and 1 tablespoon orange juice, then bake for 45 minutes with the meringues. Serve the fruit over the meringues.

roasted honey peaches

what you need

- 2 tablespoons orange blossom honey
- 1 vanilla pod, split in half lengthways
- 2-3 teaspoons sesame seeds
- 4 peaches, halved and stoned
- vanilla ice cream or half-fat crème fraîche, to serve (optional)

what you do

1. Spoon the honey into a small saucepan. Scrape the seeds from the vanilla pod and add the seeds and pod to the pan. Heat gently, stirring occasionally for 1-2 minutes. Stir in the sesame seeds.
2. Place the peaches cut side down in a roasting tin and pour over the honey mixture. Bake in a preheated oven, 180°C (350°F), Gas Mark 4, for 20-25 minutes until the peaches are soft. Baste a couple of times with the juices during cooking.
3. Serve the baked peaches warm with vanilla ice cream or crème fraîche, if liked.

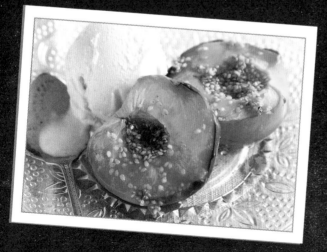

berry & mint compote

Cost
££

Timing

Serves
4

- 450 g (14½ oz) mixed fruit, such as strawberries, blackberries, raspberries and halved and stoned plums
- 1 cinnamon stick
- finely grated rind and juice of 1 orange
- 8 mint leaves, shredded
- natural yogurt, to serve (optional)

what you do

1. Place the fruit, cinnamon stick and orange rind and juice in a small saucepan and simmer gently for 12–15 minutes.
2. Remove the cinnamon stick and leave the compote to cool for 3–4 minutes, then stir in the mint.
3. Serve with dollops of natural yogurt, if liked.

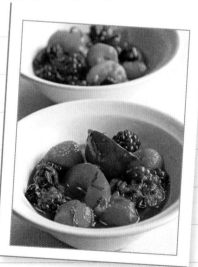

instant apple crumbles

Cost
£

Timing
⏱

Serves
4

what you do

what you need

- 1 kg (2 lb) cooking apples, such as Bramley, peeled, cored and thickly sliced
- 25 g (1 oz) butter
- 2 tablespoons caster sugar
- 1 tablespoon lemon juice
- 2 tablespoons water

Crumble
- 50 g (2 oz) butter
- 75 g (3 oz) fresh wholemeal breadcrumbs
- 25 g (1 oz) pumpkin seeds
- 2 tablespoons soft brown sugar

1. Place the apples in a saucepan with the butter, caster sugar, lemon juice and water. Cover and simmer for 8–10 minutes, until softened. Remove from the heat.
2. For the crumble, melt the butter in a frying pan, add the breadcrumbs and stir-fry over a medium heat until light golden, then add the pumpkin seeds and stir-fry for a further 1 minute. Remove from the heat and stir in the brown sugar.
3. Spoon the apple mixture into bowls, sprinkle with the crumble and serve.

Variation

For instant pear and chocolate crumbles, peel, core and slice 1 kg (2 lb) pears and cook them with the butter, caster sugar and water as above, adding ½ teaspoon ground ginger instead of the lemon juice. Prepare the crumble as above, replacing the pumpkin seeds with 50 g (2 oz) roughly chopped plain dark chocolate. Cook and serve as above.

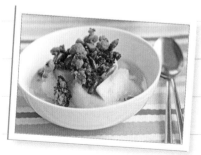

strawberry & almond layered desserts

what you need

Cost £

Timing 🕐

Serves 4

- 4 tablespoons flaked almonds
- 4 tablespoons desiccated coconut
- 300 g (10 oz) strawberries, hulled and sliced
- 250 ml (8 fl oz) natural yogurt
- 4 teaspoons clear honey

what you do

1. Place the flaked almonds and coconut on a baking sheet and cook under a preheated medium-hot grill for 3–4 minutes until golden. Give the tray a little shake at least once to ensure the almonds are lightly toasted on both sides. Leave to cool.
2. Spoon half of the almond and coconut mixture into 4 glasses. Top with half of the sliced strawberries, then all of the yogurt.
3. Top with the remaining strawberries, then the remaining almond and coconut mixture. Spoon over the honey and serve.

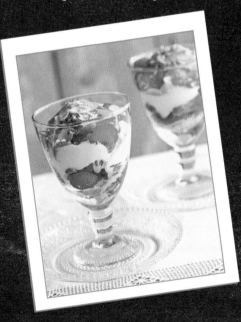

lemon & sultana rice pudding

what you need

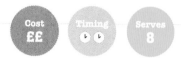

Cost
££

Timing

Serves
8

- 1 vanilla pod, split in half lengthways
- 175 g (6 oz) short-grain rice
- 750 ml (1¼ pints) milk
- 2 tablespoons sultanas
- finely grated rind of 2 lemons

- 2 teaspoons caster sugar, or to taste
- 150 ml (¼ pint) thick natural yogurt
- ground or freshly grated nutmeg, to serve

what you do

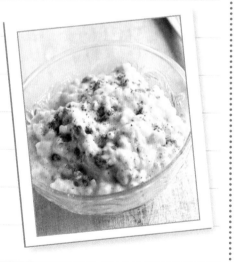

1. Scrape the seeds from the vanilla pod and add the seeds and pod to a saucepan with the rice, milk, sultanas and lemon rind.
2. Bring to the boil, then reduce the heat and simmer for 15–18 minutes, stirring occasionally, until the rice is swollen and soft. Stir in the sugar to taste and leave to cool for 10 minutes.
3. Remove the vanilla pod from the rice, then stir in the yogurt. Serve sprinkled with a little nutmeg.

warm chocolate fromage frais

Cost
£

Timing
🕐

Serves
6

what you need

- 300 g (10 oz) plain dark chocolate, broken into squares
- 500 g (1 lb) fat-free fromage frais
- 1 teaspoon vanilla extract

what you do

1. Melt the chocolate in a heatproof bowl set over a saucepan of barely simmering water, then remove from the heat. Add the fromage frais and vanilla extract and quickly stir together.
2. Divide the chocolate fromage frais between 6 little pots or glasses and serve immediately.

Variation
For warm cappuccino fromage frais, melt the plain dark chocolate with 2 tablespoons very strong (brewed) espresso coffee and then add the fat-free fromage frais. Divide between 6 espresso cups, finishing each with 1 teaspoon fromage frais and a dusting of cocoa powder.

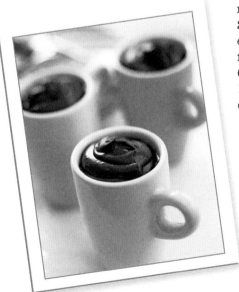

white chocolate mousse

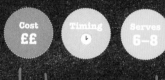

Cost ££

Timing

Serves 6–8

what you need

- 200 g (7 oz) white chocolate, chopped
- 4 tablespoons milk
- 12 cardamom pods
- 200 g (7 oz) silken tofu
- 50 g (2 oz) caster sugar
- 1 egg white
- half-fat crème fraîche or natural yogurt, to serve
- cocoa powder, for dusting

Variation

For white chocolate and amaretto pots, make the mousse mixture as above, omitting the cardamom and adding 2 tablespoons Amaretto liqueur when blending the tofu. Complete the recipe and chill as above. Serve with fresh raspberries instead of the crème fraîche or yogurt and cocoa powder.

what you do

1. Put the chocolate and milk in a heatproof bowl and melt over a saucepan of barely simmering water.
2. To release the cardamom seeds, crush the pods using a pestle and mortar. Discard the pods and crush the seeds finely. Place the crushed cardamom seeds and the tofu in a blender or food processor with half of the sugar, then blend well to make a smooth paste. Turn the mixture into a large bowl.
3. Whisk the egg white in a separate clean bowl, until it forms soft peaks. Gradually whisk in the remaining sugar.
4. Beat the melted chocolate mixture into the tofu until completely combined. Using a large metal spoon, fold in the whisked egg white.
5. Spoon the mousse into small coffee cups or glasses and chill in the fridge for at least 1 hour before serving. Serve topped with spoonfuls of crème fraîche or yogurt and a light dusting of cocoa powder.

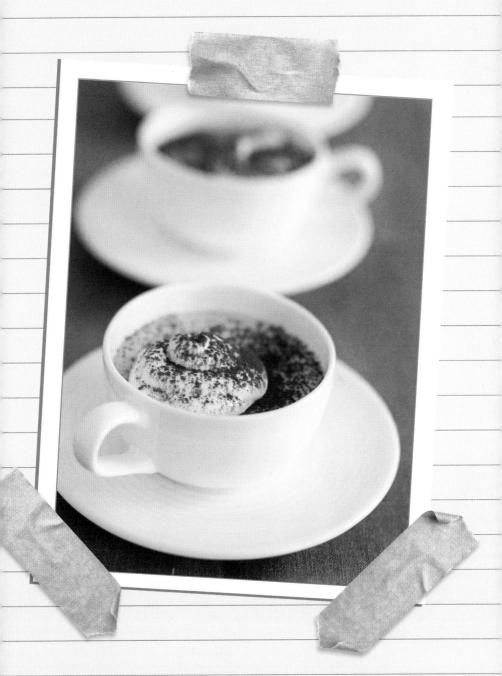

cidered apple jellies

Cost
££

Timing

Serves
6

what you need

- 1 kg (2 lb) cooking apples, peeled, cored and sliced
- 300 ml (½ pint) cider
- 150 ml (¼ pint) water, plus 4 tablespoons
- 75 g (3 oz) caster sugar
- finely grated rind of 2 lemons
- 4 teaspoons powdered gelatine
- 150 ml (¼ pint) double cream

what you do

1. Put the apples, cider, 150 ml (¼ pint) water, sugar and the rind of 1 of the lemons into a saucepan. Cover and simmer for 15 minutes until the apples are soft.
2. Meanwhile, put the remaining 4 tablespoons water into a small bowl and sprinkle over the gelatine, making sure that all the powder is absorbed by the water. Set aside.
3. Add the gelatine to the hot apples and stir until completely dissolved. Purée the apple mixture in a blender or food processor until smooth, then pour into 6 teacups or glasses. Leave to cool, then chill in the fridge for 4–5 hours until completely set.
4. When you are ready to serve, whip the cream in a bowl until it forms soft peaks. Spoon the cream over the jellies and sprinkle with the remaining lemon rind, then serve.

Variation

For cidered apple granita, omit the gelatine and pour the puréed apple mixture into a shallow dish so that the mixture is about 2.5 cm (1 inch) deep or less. Freeze for about 2 hours until mushy around the edges, then beat with a fork. Freeze for a further 2 hours, beating the granita at 30-minute intervals until it becomes the texture of crushed ice. Freeze until ready to serve, then scoop into small glasses.

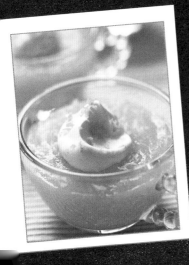

griddled bananas with blueberries

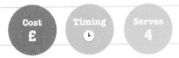

Cost £

Timing ◔

Serves 4

what you need

- 4 bananas, unpeeled
- 8 tablespoons 0%-fat Greek yogurt
- 4 tablespoons oatmeal or fine porridge oats
- 125 g (4 oz) blueberries
- clear honey, to serve

what you do

1. Heat a ridged griddle pan over a medium-high heat, add the bananas and griddle for 8–10 minutes or until the skins are beginning to blacken, turning occasionally.
2. Transfer the bananas to serving dishes and, using a sharp knife, cut open lengthways. Spoon over the yogurt and sprinkle with the oatmeal or oats and blueberries. Serve immediately, drizzled with about 1 teaspoon honey per banana.

Variation

For oatmeal, ginger and sultana yogurt, mix ½ teaspoon ground ginger with the yogurt in a bowl. Sprinkle with 2–4 tablespoons soft dark brown sugar, according to taste, the oatmeal and 4 tablespoons sultanas. Leave to stand for 5 minutes before serving.

Back to Basics

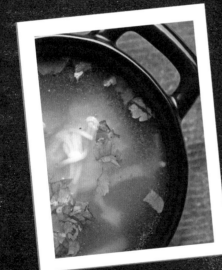

chicken stock

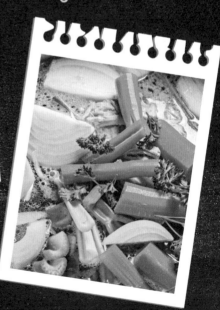

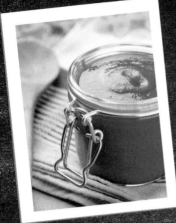

fresh tomato sauce

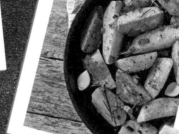

perfect roast potatoes

vegetable stock ....

gravy ....

chicken stock ....

perfect roast potatoes ....

boiled rice ....

pesto ....

fresh tomato sauce ....

béchamel sauce ....

parsley sauce ....

vegetable stock

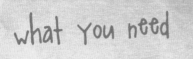

what you need

Cost £

Timing

- 1 tablespoon sunflower oil
- 2 onions, roughly chopped
- 2 carrots, roughly chopped
- 2 celery sticks, roughly chopped
- 500 g (1 lb) mixture of other prepared fresh vegetables (such as parsnips, fennel, leeks, courgettes, mushrooms and tomatoes)

- 1.5 litres (2½ pints) water
- 1 bouquet garni
- 1 teaspoon black peppercorns

what you do

1. Heat the oil in a large, heavy-based saucepan and gently fry all the vegetables for 5 minutes.
2. Add the water, bouquet garni and peppercorns, bring slowly to the boil. Reduce the heat and simmer the stock very gently for 40 minutes, skimming the surface from time to time if necessary.
3. Strain the stock through a large sieve, preferably a conical one. Don't squeeze the juice out of the vegetables or the stock will be cloudy. Leave the stock to cool completely, then chill.

gravy

what you need

- pan juices from roasted meat
- 1 tablespoon plain flour (less for a thin gravy)
- 300–400 ml (10–14 fl oz) liquid (this could be water, drained from the accompanying vegetables; stock; half stock and half water; or half wine and half water)
- salt and pepper

what you do

1. Tilt the flameproof roasting tin and skim off the fat from the surface with a large serving spoon until you are left with the pan juices and just a thin layer of fat.
2. Over a medium heat on the hob, sprinkle the flour into the tin and stir with a wooden spoon, scraping up all the residue, particularly from around the edges of the tin.
3. Gradually pour the liquid into the tin, stirring well until the gravy is thick and glossy. Let the mixture bubble, then check the seasoning, adding a little salt and pepper if necessary.

chicken stock

what you need

- 1 large chicken carcass, plus any trimmings
- giblets, except the liver, if available
- 1 onion, quartered
- 1 celery stick, roughly chopped
- 1 bouquet garni or 3 bay leaves
- 1 teaspoon black peppercorns
- 1.8 litres (3 pints) cold water

what you do

1. Put the chicken carcass, giblets, onion, celery, bouquet garni or bay leaves and peppercorns into a large, heavy-based saucepan with the water.
2. Bring slowly to the boil. Reduce the heat and simmer the stock very gently for 1½ hours, skimming the surface from time to time if necessary.
3. Strain the stock through a large sieve, preferably a conical one. Leave the stock to cool completely, then chill.

how to make perfect roast potatoes

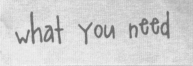

Cost
£

Timing
▶ ▶ ▶

Serves
4–6

- potatoes
- lard or sunflower oil
- sea salt

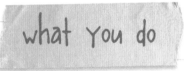

1. Peel and cut potatoes into even-sized pieces. Parboil in a saucepan of lightly salted boiling water for 10 minutes, then drain well. Shake them after draining to rough up the edges slightly.
2. Heat a roasting tin containing lard (or a good glug of sunflower oil for veggies and vegans) in a preheated oven, 220°C (425°F), Gas Mark 7, for about 5 minutes or until the lard or oil is very hot. Carefully place the potatoes in it, turning them over in the oil and then lightly sprinkle with sea salt.
3. Roast on the top shelf in the oven for 40 minutes, turning every now and then, until golden and crispy. Serve.

boiled rice

Timing

Serves
4

what you do

what you need

- 350 g (1½ oz) Thai jasmine or long-grain rice
- 300 ml (½ pint) Vegetable or Chicken Stock (see page 164–5)

1. Put the rice in a sieve and wash it under warm running water, rubbing the grains together between your hands to get rid of any excess starch.
2. Put the rice into a saucepan and add the stock. Set the pan on the smallest ring on the hob and bring it to the boil. Give it a quick stir, then reduce the heat to a simmer. Cover with a lid and leave to cook for 15 minutes.
3. Turn off the heat and allow the rice to steam with the lid on for another 20 minutes. Don't be tempted to lift the lid to check what's going on.
4. To serve, fluff up the grains of rice with a spoon or fork.

pesto

what you need

Cost
££

Timing

Serves
4

- 50 g (2 oz) fresh basil, including stalks
- 50 g (2 oz) pine nuts
- 65 g (2½ oz) grated Parmesan-style cheese
- 2 garlic cloves, chopped
- 125 ml (4 fl oz) olive oil
- salt and pepper

what you do

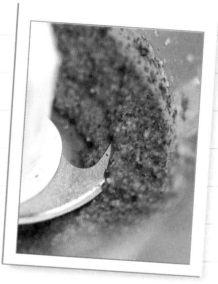

1. Tear the basil into pieces and put it into a blender or food processor with the pine nuts, cheese and garlic.
2. Process lightly until the nuts are broken into small pieces, scraping the mixture down from the sides of the bowl if necessary.
3. Add the oil and a little salt and pepper and blend to form a thick paste. Stir into freshly cooked pasta or turn into a bowl, cover and refrigerate. It can be kept, covered, for up to 5 days.

Variation

To make red pesto, drain 125 g (4 oz) sun-dried tomatoes in oil, chop them into small pieces and add to the food processor instead of the basil.

fresh tomato sauce

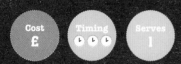

Cost £

Timing

Serves 1

what you need

- 1 kg (2 lb) very ripe, full-flavoured tomatoes
- 100 ml (3 ½ fl oz) olive oil
- 1 onion, finely chopped
- 2 garlic cloves, crushed
- 2 tablespoons chopped oregano
- sprinkling of caster sugar (optional)
- salt and pepper

TIP

This is a good sauce to make in large quantities if you have a glut of tomatoes and can be frozen in small polythene freezer bags or plastic containers.

what you do

1. Put the tomatoes in a heatproof bowl, cover with boiling water and leave for about 2 minutes or until the skins start to split. Pour away the water. Skin and roughly chop the tomatoes.
2. Heat the oil in a large, heavy-based saucepan and gently fry the onion for 5 minutes or until softened but not browned. Add the garlic and fry for a further 1 minute.
3. Add the tomatoes and cook, stirring frequently, for 20–25 minutes or until the sauce is thickened and pulpy.
4. Stir in the oregano and season to taste with salt and pepper. If the sauce is very sharp, add a sprinkling of caster sugar, if liked.

Variation
Canned tomatoes make a good alternative if the only fresh ones available don't look very appetizing. Substitute two 400 g (13 oz) cans of chopped tomatoes and cook until pulpy.

béchamel sauce

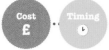

Cost £

Timing 🕐

what you do

1. Melt the butter over a medium heat in a small, heavy-based saucepan. Stir in the flour and cook gently for 1–2 minutes, stirring to make a smooth paste.
2. Remove the pan from the heat and add the milk (very gradually to avoid lumps forming), continuously whisking or beating well with a wooden spoon. When all the milk is combined you should have a smooth sauce.
3. Stir in the cream or additional milk, a little nutmeg and salt and pepper and then return the pan to the heat. Cook gently, stirring well, for about 2 minutes until the sauce is smooth and thickened. Serve immediately.

what you need

- 50 g (2 oz) butter
- 40 g (1½ oz) plain flour
- 300 ml (½ pint) milk
- 300 ml (½ pint) single cream or use 600 ml (1 pint) milk in total and omit the cream
- freshly grated nutmeg, to taste
- salt and pepper

parsley sauce

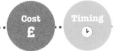

what you need

- 15 g (½ oz) parsley (choose really fresh, fragrant parsley)
- 250 ml (8 fl oz) Vegetable Stock (see page 164), fish stock or ham stock
- 25 g (1 oz) butter
- 25 g (1 oz) plain flour
- 250 ml (8 fl oz) milk
- 3 tablespoons single cream
- salt and pepper

what you do

1. Discard any tough stalks from the parsley and put it into a blender or food processor or blender with half of the stock. Blend until the parsley is very finely chopped.
2. Melt the butter over a medium heat in a heavy-based saucepan until bubbling. Tip in the flour and stir quickly to combine. Cook the mixture gently, stirring constantly with a wooden spoon, for 2 minutes.
3. Remove the pan from the heat and gradually whisk in the parsley-flavoured stock, then the remaining stock, until smooth. Whisk in the milk. Return to the heat and bring to the boil, stirring. Season with salt and pepper. Reduce the heat and continue to cook the sauce for about 5 minutes, stirring frequently, until it is smooth and glossy. The sauce should thinly coat the back of the spoon.
4. Stir in the cream and a little salt and pepper (remembering that if you've used ham stock, it might already be quite salty) and heat gently to warm through.

Index

alcohol 10, 91
almonds
  breakfast smoothie 14
  coronation chicken 118
  easy almond macaroons 146
  porridge with prune compote 28
  scribbled chocolate macaroons 146
  strawberry & almond layered
  desserts 155
apples
  apple & yoghurt muesli 23
  cidered apple granita 160
  cidered apple jellies 160
  crab, apple & avocado
  salad 121
  gingered apple & carrot
  juice 18
  instant apple crumbles 154
  one pan spiced pork 91
  pork & apple balls 36
asparagus
  prawn, potato & asparagus salad 123
aubergines
  aubergine cannelloni 50
  quick one pot ratatouille 124
  red salmon & roasted
  vegetables 103
  roasted vegetable couscous
  salad 110
  warm chicken, med veg &
  bulgar wheat salad 84
avocados 17
  avocado & banana smoothie 17
  brainfood bowl 116
  chicken fajitas with no chilli
  sauce 80
  crab, apple & avocado salad 121
  goats' cheese & spinach
  quesadillas 125
  guacamole 128
  turkey & avocado salad 121

bacon
  spaghetti carbonara 51
  squash & broccoli soup 49
  steak meatloaf 87
  sweet potato & cabbage soup 49
bananas
  avocado & banana smoothie 17
  banana & peanut butter 15
  banana & sultana drop scones 26
  breakfast smoothie 14
  griddled bananas with
  blueberries 161
  mixed grain porridge 25
  sweet quinoa porridge with banana
  and dates 28
basil
  pesto 168
beans
  broccoli & black eyed bean
  curry 68
  butter bean & chorizo stew 95
  Caribbean chicken with rice &
  peas 73
  cheesy squash, pepper & mixed
  bean soup 48
  garlic prawns with butter beans 95
  garlicky pork with warm butter

bean salad 90
  hearty minestrone 42
  mixed bean & tomato chilli 67
  mixed bean salad 122
  salmon with green vegetables 56
  spicy sausage bake 92
  squash, kale & mixed bean soup 48
  sweet potato & bean `steamed
  buns' 37
  tuna & borlotti bean salad 122
  West Indian beef & bean stew 96
béchamel sauce 170
beef
  beef & barley brö 46
  beef, pumpkin & prune stew 97
  bolognese sauce 53
  steak meatloaf 87
  Swedish meatballs 86
  West Indian beef & bean stew 96
beetroot
  falafels with beetroot salad & mint
  yoghurt 33
berries
  berry & mint compote 153
  berry, honey & yoghurt pots 21
  summer berry drop scones 26
bhajis, salmon & rice 131
blackcurrant polenta mug
  cake 141
blackened tofu wraps 39
blueberries
  blueberry, oat & honey crumble 22
  griddled bananas with
  blueberries 161
  wholemeal blueberry pancakes
  with lemon curd yoghurt 29
bolognese sauce 53
brainfood bowl 116
breadcrumbs 31
breakfast smoothie 14
broccoli
  brainfood bowl 116
  broccoli & black eyed bean curry 68
  macaroni cheese surprise 59
  smoked mackerel superfood
  salad 114
  squash and broccoli soup 49
buckwheat
  mixed grain porridge 25
budgeting 6
bulgar wheat
  warm chicken, med veg & bulgar
  wheat salad 84
butternut squash
  barley & ginger risotto with
  butternut squash 65
  butternut & rosemary soup 47
  butternut squash & ricotta
  frittata 63
  cheesy squash, pepper and mixed
  bean soup 48
  one pan spiced pork 91
  smoked mackerel superfood
  salad 114
  spinach & butternut
  lasagne 61
  squash and broccoli soup 49
  squash, kale & mixed bean soup 48
cabbage
  chilli cabbage 133
  roast pork loin with creamy
  cabbage & leeks 88

sweet potato & cabbage soup 49
cakes
  blackcurrant polenta mug
  cake 141
  chocolate, courgette & nut
  cake 144
  courgette, lemon & poppy seed
  cake 140
  gluten free coconut & mango
  cake 143
  lemon drizzle cake 145
  spiced passion mug cake 142
carbohydrates 11
Caribbean chicken with rice & peas 73
carrots
  beef & barley brö 46
  gingered apple & carrot juice 18
  macaroni cheese surprise 59
  red pepper and carrot soup 45
  spiced passion mug cake 142
  vegetable stock 164
cauliflower
  cauliflower & chickpea curry 68
  Massaman lentils with
  cauliflower 107
  vegetable, fruit & nut biryani 71
cheese
  aubergine cannelloni 50
  barley & ginger risotto with
  butternut squash 65
  butternut squash & ricotta
  frittata 63
  cheesy pork with parsnip
  purée 93
  cheesy squash, pepper &
  mixed bean soup 48
  courgette & ricotta bakes 137
  courgette, feta & mint salad 115
  goats' cheese & spinach
  quesadillas 125
  Greek salad with toasted
  pitta 112
  lemon & herb risotto 66
  macaroni cheese surprise 59
  mushroom & rocket seeded
  wrap with feta & garlic
  dressing 38
  mushrooms stuffed with courgettes
  and ricotta 137
  oven baked turkey & gruyère
  burgers 85
  pesto 168
  quick tuna fishcakes 102
  roasted vegetable couscous salad 110
  smoked mackerel & chive pâté 126
  spaghetti carbonara 51
  spicy sausage bake 92
  spinach & butternut lasagne 61
  spinach & potato tortilla 62
chicken
  Caribbean chicken with rice &
peas 73
  chicken & spinach stew 74
  chicken with breaded tomato
topping 93
  chicken burgers with tomato
  salsa 79
  chicken fajitas with no chilli sauce 80
  chicken jalfrezi 76
  chicken shawarma 77
  chicken stock 165
  chilli & coriander chicken burgers
  with mango salsa 79

coronation chicken 118
pot roast chicken 81
roasted lemony chicken with courgettes 82
spiced chicken & mango salad 118
tandoori chicken salad 120
warm chicken, med veg & bulgar wheat salad 84
chickpeas
cauliflower & chickpea curry 68
falafel pitta pockets 32
falafels with beetroot salad & mint yoghurt 33
hot & smoky hummus with warm flatbread 127
chillies
chicken jalfrezi 76
chilli & coriander chicken burgers with mango salsa 79
chilli cabbage 133
chilli kale 133
fried rice with Chinese leaves and chilli 132
ranch style eggs 60
soy tofu salad with coriander 117
tuna & borlotti bean salad 122
Chinese leaves
fried rice with Chinese leaves and chilli 132
chocolate 11
chocolate peanut cookies 147
instant pear and chocolate crumbles 154
plain dark chocolate and ginger cookies 148
scribbled chocolate macaroons 146
warm chocolate fromage frais 157
white chocolate & Amaretto pots 158
white chocolate mousse 158
chocolate, courgette & nut cake 144
chorizo
butter bean & chorizo stew 95
chorizo & ham eggs 94
jambalaya with chorizo & peppers 78
cider
cidered apple granita 160
cidered apple jellies 160
coconut
gluten free coconut & mango cake 143
strawberry & almond layered desserts 155
coconut milk
Caribbean chicken with rice & peas 73
coconut noodles in a mug 106
cod
baked cod with tomatoes & olives 98
steamed cod with lemon 98
cookies
chocolate peanut cookies 147
cranberry & hazelnut cookies 148
plain dark chocolate and ginger cookies 148
cooking times 11
coriander
chicken fajitas with no chilli sauce 80
chilli & coriander chicken burgers with mango salsa 79
falafel pitta pockets 52

goats' cheese & spinach quesadillas 125
soy tofu salad with coriander 117
coronation chicken 118
courgettes
chocolate, courgette & nut cake 144
coconut noodles in a mug 106
courgette & ricotta bakes 137
courgette, feta & mint salad 115
courgette, lemon & poppy seed cake 140
lemon & herb risotto 66
mushrooms stuffed with courgettes and ricotta 137
quick one pot ratatouille 124
red pepper and courgette soup 45
roasted lemony chicken with courgettes 82
roasted vegetable couscous salad 110
spicy courgette fritters 130
sweet potato & bean `steamed buns' 37
warm chicken, med veg & bulgar wheat salad 84
couscous
roasted vegetable couscous salad 110
rocket & cucumber couscous 103
crab
crab & grapefruit salad 123
crab, apple & avocado salad 121
cranberry & hazelnut cookies 148
cranberry sauce
Swedish meatballs 86
crème fraîche
white chocolate mousse 158
cucumber
cucumber lassi 19
fattoush salad 111
quick curried egg salad 109
rocket & cucumber couscous 103
salmon & rice bhajis 131
spiced chicken & mango salad 118
curries
broccoli & black eyed bean curry 68
cauliflower & chickpea curry 68
chicken jalfrezi 76
vegetable curry with rice 70

dates
sweet quinoa porridge with banana and dates 28
drop scones 26

eggs
butternut squash & ricotta frittata 63
chorizo & ham eggs 94
courgette & ricotta bakes 137
haddock with poached eggs 100
light egg fried rice 132
linguine with shredded ham & eggs 52
quick curried egg salad 109
ranch style eggs 60
smoked mackerel kedgeree 101
spaghetti carbonara 51
spinach & potato tortilla 62
equipment 8 9

falafel pitta pockets 32
falafels with beetroot salad & mint yoghurt 33
fattoush salad 111
fish

oily 11
omega 3 rich 126
fizzy drinks 10, 112
flatbreads
hot & smoky hummus with warm flatbread 127
flour tortillas
chicken fajitas with no chilli sauce 80
goats' cheese & spinach quesadillas 125
food labelling 10
food poisoning 78
freezers 8, 101
fromage frais
warm chocolate fromage frais 157
fruit 9, 19
maple glazed granola with fruit 24

garlic
butter bean & chorizo stew 95
garlic prawns with butter beans 95
garlicky pork with warm butter bean salad 90
pot roast chicken 81
roasted lemony chicken with courgettes 82
ginger
barley & ginger risotto with butternut squash 65
gingered apple & carrot juice 18
oatmeal, ginger & sultana yoghurt 161
plain dark chocolate and ginger cookies 148
spiced passion mug cake 142
gluten free coconut & mango cake 143
goats' cheese & spinach quesadillas 125
granola
berry, honey & yoghurt pots 21
maple glazed granola with fruit 24
on the go granola breakfast bars 30
grapefruit
brainfood bowl 116
crab & grapefruit salad 123
gravy 165
Greek salad with toasted pitta 112
green tea 11
guacamole 128

ham
chorizo & ham eggs 94
linguine with shredded ham & eggs 52
hazelnuts
brainfood bowl 116
chocolate, courgette & nut cake 144
cranberry & hazelnut cookies 148
healthy habits 10 11
herbs
chunky summer vegetable soup with mixed herb gremolata 44
healthy mashed potatoes 136
lemon & herb risotto 66
honey
blueberry, oat & honey crumble 22
brainfood bowl 116
chocolate peanut cookies 147
griddled bananas with blueberries 161
one pan spiced pork 91
roasted honey peaches 152
spiced passion mug cake 142
strawberry & almond layered desserts 155

internet shopping 7

kale
   chilli kale 133
   squash, kale & mixed bean soup 48
kedgeree style rice with spinach 64

leeks
   macaroni cheese surprise 59
   roast pork loin with creamy
   cabbage & leeks 88
   salmon with green vegetables 56
lemon curd
   courgette, lemon & poppy seed
   cake 140
   wholemeal blueberry pancakes
   with lemon curd yoghurt 29
lemons
   cidered apple jellies 160
   courgette, lemon & poppy seed
   cake 140
   lemon & sultana rice pudding 156
   lemon drizzle cake 145
   roasted lemony chicken with
   courgettes 82
   steamed cod with lemon 98
lentils
   butternut & rosemary soup 47
   chicken & spinach stew 74
   Massaman lentils with cauliflower 107
   pot roast chicken 81
lettuce
   chicken shawarma 77
   fattoush salad 111
   quick curried egg salad 109
limes
   Caribbean chicken with rice & peas 73
   chilli kale 133
   goats' cheese & spinach
   quesadillas 125
   quick curried egg salad 109
linguine with shredded ham & eggs 52

macaroons 146
mackerel 126
   see also smoked mackerel
mangoes
   chilli & coriander chicken
   burgers with mango salsa 79
   gluten free coconut & mango
   cake 143
   mango & orange smoothie 16
   mango & passion fruit trifle 150
   mango lassi 16
   maple glazed granola with fruit 24
   spiced chicken & mango salad 118
   maple glazed granola with fruit 24
markets 7
Massaman lentils with cauliflower 107
meal planner 8
meringue 151
millet
   mixed grain porridge 25
mint
   berry & mint compote 153
   courgette, feta & mint salad 115
   Greek salad with toasted pitta 112
   salmon & rice bhajis 131
   spicy courgette fritters 130
mood boosters 11
muesli, apple & yoghurt 23
mushrooms
   mushroom & rocket seeded wrap
   with feta & garlic dressing 38
   mushrooms stuffed with courgettes
   and ricotta 137

nectarines
   baked nectarines with orange
   meringues 151
nuts 34

oats
   blueberry, oat & honey crumble 22
   breakfast smoothie 14
   cranberry & hazelnut cookies 148
   griddled bananas with blueberries 161
   maple glazed granola with fruit 24
   oatmeal, ginger & sultana yoghurt 161
   porridge with prune compote 28
oily fish 11
olives
   baked cod with tomatoes & olives 98
   Greek salad with toasted pitta 112
   red salmon & roasted vegetables 103
   tuna & olive pasta 55
omega 3 rich fish 126
orange juice
   mango & orange smoothie 16
oranges
   baked nectarines with orange
   meringues 151
   berry & mint compote 153
   chocolate, courgette & nut cake 144

pancakes
   wholemeal blueberry pancakes
   with lemon curd yoghurt 29
pancetta
   spaghetti carbonara 51
parsnips
   one pan spiced pork 91
parsley
   chunky summer vegetable soup
   with mixed herb gremolata 44
   parsley sauce 171
   potato wedges with yoghurt &
   parsley dip 135
parsnips
   cheesy pork with parsnip purée 93
passion fruit
   mango & passion fruit trifle 150
pasta
   aubergine cannelloni 50
   hearty minestrone 42
   linguine with shredded ham &
   eggs 52
   macaroni cheese surprise 59
   spaghetti carbonara 51
   spicy sausage bake 92
   spinach & butternut lasagne 61
   tuna & olive pasta 55
   tuna layered lasagne 54
   wholemeal 59
peaches
   roasted honey peaches 152
peanut butter
   banana & peanut butter 15
   chocolate peanut cookies 147
peanuts
   brown rice salad with peanuts &
   raisins 34
pearl barley
   barley & ginger risotto with
   butternut squash 65
   beef & barley brö 46
pears
   instant pear and chocolate
   crumbles 154
peas

kedgeree style rice with spinach 64
   salmon with green
   vegetables 56
   smoked mackerel superfood
   salad 114
pedometers 128
peppers
   broccoli & black eyed bean
   curry 68
   butter bean & chorizo stew 95
   cauliflower & chickpea curry 68
   chicken jalfrezi 76
   chorizo & ham eggs 94
   jambalaya with chorizo & peppers 78
   potato wedges with yoghurt &
   parsley dip 135
   quick one pot ratatouille 124
   ranch style eggs 60
   red pepper and carrot soup 45
   red pepper and courgette soup 45
   red salmon & roasted vegetables 103
   roasted vegetable couscous salad 110
   spinach & potato tortilla 62
   steak meatloaf 87
   tuna & jalapeño baked potatoes 58
   warm chicken, med veg & bulgar
   wheat salad 84
pesto 168
   chicken burgers with tomato salsa 79
pine nuts
   pesto 168
   quick spinach with pine nuts 134
   roasted vegetable couscous salad 110
pineapple
   spiced passion mug cake 142
pitta bread
   chicken shawarma 77
   falafel pitta pockets 32
   fattoush salad 111
   Greek salad with toasted pitta 112
   sweet potato & bean
   steamed buns' 37
polenta
   blackcurrant polenta mug cake 141
pomegranate juice
   breakfast smoothie 14
pomegranate seeds
   roasted vegetable couscous salad 110
popping corn 149
poppy seeds
   courgette, lemon & poppy seed
   cake 140
pork
   cheesy pork with parsnip purée 93
   garlicky pork with warm butter
   bean salad 90
   one pan spiced pork 91
   pork & apple balls 36
   roast pork loin with creamy
   cabbage & leeks 88
   steak meatloaf 87
   Swedish meatballs 86
porridge
   mixed grain porridge 25
   porridge with prune compote 28
   sweet quinoa porridge with banana
   and dates 27
potatoes
   haddock with poached eggs 100
   healthy mashed potatoes 136
   perfect roast potatoes 166
   potato wedges with yoghurt &
   parsley dip 135
   prawn, potato & asparagus salad 123

quick tuna fishcakes 102
spinach & potato tortilla 62
summer vegetable soup 44
tuna & jalapeño baked potatoes 58
prawns
    garlic prawns with butter beans 95
    prawn, potato & asparagus salad 123
preparation times 11
prunes
    beef, pumpkin & prune stew 97
    porridge with prune compote 28
pumpkin
    beef, pumpkin & prune stew 97
pumpkin seeds
    brainfood bowl 116
    instant apple crumbles 154
    on the go granola breakfast bars 30

quinoa
    mixed grain porridge 25
    smoked mackerel superfood
    salad 114
    sweet quinoa porridge with banana
    and dates 28

raisins
    brown rice salad with peanuts &
    raisins 34
    chicken & spinach stew 74
    on the go granola breakfast bars 30
ranch style eggs 60
raspberries
    white chocolate & Amaretto pots 158
ratatouille, quick one pot 124
red pesto 168
rice
    boiled rice 167
    brainfood bowl 116
    brown rice salad with peanuts &
    raisins 34
    Caribbean chicken with rice &
    peas 73
    fried rice with Chinese leaves and
    chilli 132
    jambalaya with chorizo & peppers 78
    kedgeree style rice with spinach 64
    lemon & herb risotto 66
    lemon & sultana rice pudding 156
    light egg fried rice 132
    salmon & rice bhajis 131
    smoked mackerel kedgeree 101
    vegetable curry with rice 70
    vegetable, fruit & nut biryani 71
rice noodles
    coconut noodles in a mug 106
rocket
    crab & grapefruit salad 123
    garlic prawns with butter beans 95
    mushroom & rocket seeded wrap
    with feta & garlic dressing 38
    rocket & cucumber couscous 103
    tuna & borlotti bean salad 122
rosemary
    butternut & rosemary soup 47

sage
    butternut squash & ricotta
    frittata 63
    cheesy pork with parsnip purée 93
salad leaves
    tandoori chicken salad 120
    turkey & avocado salad 121
salmon
    red salmon & roasted vegetables 103

salmon & rice bhajis 131
salmon with green vegetables 56
sausages
    spicy sausage bake 92
scribbled chocolate macaroons 146
seeded spelt soda bread 31
seeded wraps
    blackened tofu wraps 39
    mushroom & rocket seeded wrap
    with feta & garlic dressing 38
seeds 34
sesame seeds
    hot & smoky hummus with warm
    flatbread 127
    on the go granola breakfast bars 30
    roasted honey peaches 152
    seeded spelt soda bread 51
shopping for food 6 7, 101
smoked haddock
    haddock with poached eggs 100
    kedgeree style rice with spinach 64
smoked mackerel
    smoked mackerel & chive pâté 126
    smoked mackerel kedgeree 101
    smoked mackerel superfood
    salad 114
smoothies 19
    avocado & banana smoothie 17
    breakfast smoothie 14
    mango & orange smoothie 16
snacks 109
    nuts 34
soda bread, seeded spelt 31
soups
    beef & barley brö 46
    butternut & rosemary soup 47
    cheesy squash, pepper and mixed
    bean soup 48
    chunky summer vegetable soup
    with mixed herb gremolata 44
    hearty minestrone 42
    red pepper and carrot soup 45
    red pepper and courgette soup 45
    squash and broccoli soup 49
    squash, kale & mixed bean soup 48
    summer vegetable soup 44
    sweet potato & cabbage soup 49
soy tofu salad with coriander 117
soya milk 25
spinach
    chicken & spinach stew 74
    chorizo & ham eggs 94
    goats' cheese & spinach
    quesadillas 125
    hearty minestrone 42
    kedgeree style rice with spinach 64
    quick spinach with pine nuts 134
    spinach & butternut lasagne 61
    spinach & potato tortilla 62
spring onions
    linguine with shredded ham &
    eggs 52
steak meatloaf 87
stock
    chicken 165
    vegetable 164
storecupboard essentials 7 8
strawberries
    baked strawberries & meringue 151
    strawberry & almond layered
    desserts 155
    watermelon cooler 18
sugar 10
sugar snap peas

brainfood bowl 116
sultanas
    banana & sultana drop scones 26
    coronation chicken 118
    lemon & sultana rice pudding 156
    oatmeal, ginger & sultana
    yoghurt 161
    vegetable, fruit & nut biryani 71
summer vegetable soup 44
supermarket bargains 101
swede
    beef & barley brö 46
Swedish meatballs 86
sweet potatoes
    baked sweet potatoes 72
    roast pork loin with creamy
    cabbage & leeks 88
    sweet potato & bean `steamed
    buns' 37
    sweet potato & cabbage soup 49
    vegetable, fruit & nut biryani 71
sweetcorn
    Caribbean chicken with rice &
    peas 73

tahini 15
    chicken shawarma 77
tandoori chicken salad 120
tea, green 11
Thai basil
    Massaman lentils with
    cauliflower 107
toffee & chocolate popcorn 149
toffee, marshmallow & nut popcorn 149
tofu
    blackened tofu wraps 39
    soy tofu salad with coriander 117
    steamed chilli soy tofu 117
    white chocolate mousse 158
tomatoes
    aubergine cannelloni 50
    baked cod with tomatoes & olives 98
    bolognese sauce 53
    butter bean & chorizo stew 95
    cauliflower & chickpea curry 68
    chicken with breaded tomato
    topping 93
    chicken burgers with tomato salsa 79
    chicken jalfrezi 76
    chorizo & ham eggs 94
    fattoush salad 111
    fresh tomato sauce 169
    garlicky pork with warm butter
    bean salad 90
    goats' cheese & spinach
    quesadillas 125
    Greek salad with toasted pitta 112
    guacamole 128
    mixed bean & tomato chilli 67
    quick curried egg salad 109
    quick one pot ratatouille 124
    quick spinach with pine nuts 134
    ranch style eggs 60
    red pesto 168
    spicy sausage bake 92
    spinach & butternut lasagne 61
    tuna & olive pasta 55
    tuna layered lasagne 54
tuna
    quick tuna fishcakes 102
    tuna & borlotti bean salad 122
    tuna & jalapeño baked potatoes 58
    tuna & olive pasta 55
    tuna layered lasagne 54

turkey
    oven baked turkey & gruyère
    burgers 85
    turkey & avocado salad 121
use by dates 78
vanilla
    lemon & sultana rice pudding 156
    warm chocolate fromage frais 157
veal
    Swedish meatballs 86
vegetables 9
    roasted vegetable couscous salad 110
    salmon with green vegetables 56
    summer vegetable soup 44
    vegetable curry with rice 70
    vegetable, fruit & nut biryani 71
    vegetable stock 164
    warm chicken, med veg & bulgar
    wheat salad 84
walnuts
    oven baked turkey & gruyère
    burgers 85
water 11, 14, 42
watercress
    crab & grapefruit salad 123
    haddock with poached eggs 100
    spiced chicken & mango salad 118
watermelon cooler 18
West Indian beef & bean stew 96
white chocolate mousse 158

yoghurt
    apple & yoghurt muesli 23
    berry, honey & yoghurt pots 21
    chicken jalfrezi 76
    coronation chicken 118
    courgette, lemon & poppy seed
    cake 140
    cucumber lassi 19
    falafels with beetroot salad & mint
    yoghurt 33
    griddled bananas with
    blueberries 161
    mango & orange smoothie 16
    mango & passion fruit trifle 150
    mango lassi 16
    maple glazed granola with fruit 24
    mixed grain porridge 25
    oatmeal, ginger & sultana
    yoghurt 161
    potato wedges with yoghurt &
    parsley dip 135
    quick curried egg salad 109
    salmon & rice bhajis 131
    soya yoghurt 25
    spiced chicken & mango salad 118
    strawberry & almond layered
    desserts 155
    tandoori chicken salad 120
    wholemeal blueberry pancakes
    with lemon curd yoghurt 29

Picture Credits

Dreamstime.com All1962 163 left; Sergii Koval 163 right; Zigzagmtart 162 right. **istockphoto.com** joannawnuk 162 left. **Octopus Publishing Group** David Munns 138 left, 149, 157; Gareth Sambidge 19; Ian Wallace 32, 72, 99; Lis Parsons 14, 22, 23, 29, 54, 63, 73, 76, 83, 84, 89, 90, 93, 94, 97, 104 right, 115, 121, 123, 125, 129, 131, 138 right, 141, 142, 152, 153, 155, 156; Stephen Conroy 9, 50, 51, 52, 53, 57, 71, 86, 87, 92, 124, 168; Will Heap 4, 12 right, 20, 40, 43, 62, 67, 69, 75, 104 left, 108, 111, 113, 132, 154; William Lingwood 119; William Reavell 30, 35, 36, 64, 133; William Shaw 12 left, 16, 24, 27, 46, 49, 55, 117, 146, 159, 160. **Shutterstock** inxti 5; Picsfive 3; Pinkyone 2; piotr_pabijan 6; STILLFX 12; The_Pixel 8; Utro_na_more 9 background.